30 MINUTE THYROID COOKBOOK FOR BEGINNERS

Quick and Easy Recipes for Managing Hypothyroidism and Hyperthyroidism, Offering Nutritional Support for Balanced Thyroid Function in 30 Minutes

Kingsley Klopp

As a token of our gratitude for your purchasing our book, we will be providing you with extra bonuses.

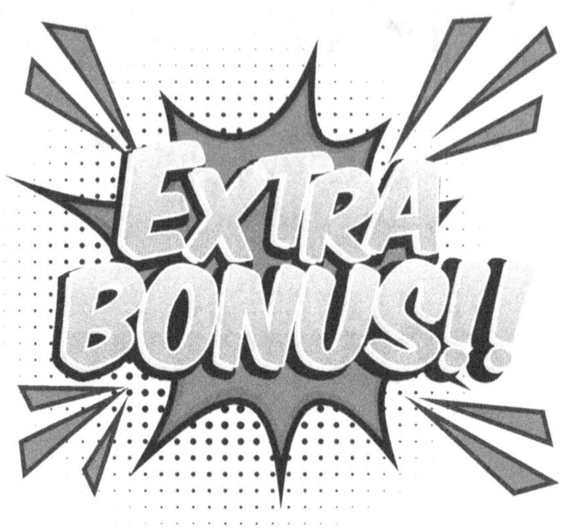

1. **WEEKLY MEAL PLANNER JOURNAL**
2. **FREE E-BOOK FEATURING FULL-COLOR IMAGES OF THE FINISHED RECIPES.**

Table of Contents

Fish & Seafood Recipes

Special Note

We understand that managing thyroid health can be complex and deeply personal, and this cookbook is here to support you every step of the way. As you set out on your gastronomic adventure, we encourage you to remember that individual dietary needs can vary significantly. While these recipes are crafted to support thyroid health broadly, your unique condition may require specific adjustments. We recommend using these recipes as a foundation, a starting point from which you can tailor ingredients and portions to fit your personal health requirements.

Please consider this book as your companion in the kitchen—a guide to help you navigate your diet with more ease and enjoyment. However, it's important to consult with your healthcare provider if you find yourself unsure about how best to adapt your diet to your thyroid condition. They can offer personalized advice that complements the nutritional guidance provided here.

We also want to note that the nutritional information accompanying each recipe is approximate. Variations in ingredient choices and sizes mean that these figures can change. We encourage you to think of these numbers as a guideline rather than an exact science, giving you the flexibility to adjust recipes according to what's available in your pantry and what feels right for your body.

Additionally, if this cookbook has enhanced your cooking and dining experience, we would love to read about your journey in an Amazon review. Conversely, if you encounter any issues with the recipes, please feel free to reach out to us at **kloppkingsley@gmail.com.** We are dedicated to assisting you throughout your culinary adventure.

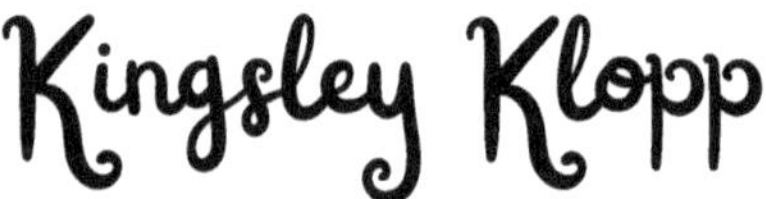

Introduction

Welcome to the **"30 Minute Thyroid Cookbook for Beginners,"** a book that promises not just to guide you through the basics of thyroid-friendly cooking, but to transform your meals into moments of healing, pleasure, and discovery. If you're stepping into these pages, you may be grappling with thyroid issues yourself or caring for someone who is. It's a journey that can feel a bit daunting at first—after all, your diet now plays a pivotal role in your health and well-being. Thyroid disorders can turn the body's own systems into something of a mystery. Whether you're dealing with hypothyroidism, hyperthyroidism, or autoimmune conditions like Hashimoto's disease, you know that what you eat matters significantly. But here's the hopeful news: mastering the right diet can be your most powerful tool in managing your thyroid health. And guess what? It doesn't require all-day prep or bland, unappealing food.

This cookbook is your friendly companion in the kitchen, designed to demystify the art of cooking for thyroid health without taking up all your time. Every recipe here can be made in 30 minutes or less—because maintaining your health shouldn't mean sacrificing all your leisure time. Imagine dishes that are not only quick to prepare but also delicious and tailored to boost your thyroid health. Ingredients rich in selenium, zinc, and iodine, balanced for optimal nutrition, come together in simple, straightforward recipes that delight the taste buds.

We know that change can be hard, especially when it comes to overhauling your diet. That's why this book emphasizes simplicity and enjoyment. It's packed with practical tips, a friendly guide to the nutrients your thyroid needs, and advice on ingredients to embrace or avoid—all presented in a way that's easy to digest and apply. As you turn these pages, you'll find more than just recipes. You'll discover stories from people just like you—people who once felt overwhelmed by their diagnosis but have since taken control of their health through the kitchen. Their journeys illuminate the path from confusion to clarity, showing how empowering cooking for thyroid health can be.

However, this book is much than just a compendium of stories and recipes. It's a toolkit, one that equips you with the knowledge to make informed, healthy choices that fit your lifestyle. Whether you're a novice in the kitchen or an experienced cook looking to tailor your meals for thyroid health, you'll find valuable insights and inspiration here.

So let's get started on this gastronomic adventure together. Let's explore new flavors, rekindle our passion for cooking, and perhaps most importantly, learn to cherish the food that nourishes not just our bodies, but also our souls. Here's to your health, one delicious, thyroid-friendly meal at a time!

Chapter 1: Understanding Your Thyroid

THE ROLE OF THE THYROID IN YOUR BODY

The thyroid gland plays a pivotal role in regulating numerous metabolic processes throughout the body. It's a small, butterfly-shaped gland located in the front of the neck, just below the Adam's apple. Despite its modest size, the thyroid has a monumental influence on overall health and well-being.

Hormone Production

The primary function of the thyroid gland is to produce, store, and release hormones into the bloodstream. The two main hormones it produces are thyroxine (T4) and triiodothyronine (T3). These hormones are crucial because they regulate the metabolism—the process by which your body converts what you eat and drink into energy.

Metabolic Rate Regulation

Thyroid hormones have a direct impact on the basal metabolic rate (BMR), which is the rate at which your body uses energy while at rest. They influence how fast your body burns calories, affecting weight loss or weight gain. A well-functioning thyroid will maintain a balanced metabolic rate, supporting various functions such as breathing, circulating blood, and regulating body temperature.

Impact on Other Systems

Thyroid hormones are integral to the development and proper functioning of many bodily systems:

- **Cardiovascular System:** Thyroid hormones increase heart rate and force of contraction, leading to an increase in blood flow and ensuring oxygen and nutrients are efficiently distributed throughout the body.
- **Digestive System:** They influence the speed at which food moves through the digestive tract, affecting bowel regularity.
- **Nervous System:** Adequate thyroid hormone levels ensure good nerve conduction and brain function.
- **Reproductive System:** Thyroid health affects reproductive hormones, which can influence menstrual regularity and fertility.

Development and Growth

Thyroid hormones are crucial for normal growth and development in infants and children. This includes not just physical stature, but also the development of the brain and nervous system. In adults, these hormones continue to play roles in maintaining organ system maturity and overall health.

Interaction with Other Hormones

The thyroid gland doesn't operate in isolation; it interacts with other glands in the endocrine system. For instance, it is regulated by the pituitary gland, which produces Thyroid Stimulating Hormone (TSH). TSH signals the thyroid to produce more T3 and T4 when levels are low, and less when they are high. Additionally, thyroid function can affect levels of sex hormones, stress hormones, and growth hormones.

Thus, the thyroid gland, through its hormone production, plays a fundamental role in managing energy use, regulating the body's metabolic rate, and ensuring the proper function of various bodily systems. This underscores why maintaining thyroid health is essential for overall bodily function and well-being. Thyroid disorders, such as hypothyroidism (underactive thyroid) or hyperthyroidism (overactive thyroid), can have profound impacts on numerous aspects of health, illustrating the critical balance the thyroid plays in human physiology.

COMMON THYROID DISORDERS: HYPOTHYROIDISM AND HYPERTHYROIDISM

Thyroid disorders are common endocrine conditions, with hypothyroidism and hyperthyroidism being the most prevalent forms. These conditions stem from the improper functioning of the thyroid gland, which can significantly impact the body's metabolic processes and overall health.

Hypothyroidism

Definition and Causes: Hypothyroidism occurs when the thyroid gland does not produce enough thyroid hormones (T3 and T4). This underactivity can result from various causes:

- **Hashimoto's thyroiditis:** An autoimmune disorder where the immune system attacks the thyroid gland.
- **Iodine deficiency:** Critical for thyroid hormone production, a lack of dietary iodine can lead to hypothyroidism.
- **Thyroidectomy:** Surgical removal of all or part of the thyroid gland can result in decreased hormone production.
- **Radiation therapy:** Used to treat cancers of the head and neck, this can damage the thyroid gland.
- **Certain medications:** Lithium and some other medications can impact thyroid hormone production.

Symptoms: The deficiency in thyroid hormone levels leads to a slowdown in the body's metabolic processes. Symptoms typically develop slowly and can include:

- Fatigue and lethargy
- Increased sensitivity to cold
- Constipation
- Dry skin and hair loss
- Weight gain
- Puffy face
- Hoarseness
- Muscle weakness and aches
- Depression
- Impaired memory

Diagnosis and Treatment: Diagnosis of hypothyroidism is primarily based on symptoms and confirmed through blood tests that measure levels of TSH and free T4. Treatment typically involves daily use of the synthetic thyroid hormone levothyroxine, which restores adequate hormone levels, reversing the symptoms and normalizing body metabolism.

Hyperthyroidism

Definition and Causes: Hyperthyroidism is the condition of having an overactive thyroid gland, producing excessive amounts of thyroid hormones. Key causes include:

- **Graves' disease:** The most common cause, this is an autoimmune disorder where the immune system stimulates the thyroid to produce too much hormone.
- **Toxic adenomas:** Nodules develop in the thyroid gland and begin to secrete thyroid hormones, upsetting the body's chemical balance.
- **Subacute thyroiditis:** Inflammation of the thyroid that causes the gland to leak excess hormones, resulting in temporary hyperthyroidism that may last a few weeks but could persist longer.
- **Excessive iodine:** A key ingredient in T3 and T4, an excess can lead to hyperthyroidism especially in individuals with pre-existing thyroid problems.

Symptoms: Hyperthyroidism leads to a generalized speeding up of metabolic processes, which can manifest as:

- Unexpected weight loss, even when appetite and food intake increase
- Rapid or irregular heartbeat (tachycardia) or palpitations
- Nervousness, anxiety, and irritability
- Tremors (fine shaking in hands or fingers)
- Sweating
- Changes in menstrual patterns
- Increased sensitivity to heat
- More frequent bowel movements
- Enlarged thyroid gland (goiter)
- Fatigue, muscle weakness

Diagnosis and Treatment: Like hypothyroidism, hyperthyroidism is diagnosed through symptom observation and blood tests. Treatment may include radioactive iodine to slow the production of thyroid hormones, anti-thyroid medications, beta blockers to manage symptoms, or surgery to remove part of the thyroid gland.

Managing Thyroid Health

Both hypothyroidism and hyperthyroidism are manageable with the right medical care, but they require ongoing monitoring and adjustment of treatment. Untreated, these thyroid disorders can lead to serious health issues, including heart problems, infertility, and in extreme cases, life-threatening conditions such as myxedema coma (in hypothyroidism) or thyroid storm (in hyperthyroidism).

HOW DIET INFLUENCES THYROID HEALTH

The diet plays a crucial role in thyroid health by affecting how the thyroid functions and how thyroid hormone levels are regulated within the body. Various nutrients directly impact thyroid function, and eating a well-balanced diet can help maintain thyroid health or manage thyroid disorders.

Key Nutrients for Thyroid Function
Iodine: Iodine is critical for the synthesis of thyroid hormones, as it is a major component of both thyroxine (T4) and triiodothyronine (T3). An iodine deficiency can lead to decreased production of these hormones, resulting in hypothyroidism, while excessive iodine intake can sometimes trigger hyperthyroidism or exacerbate existing thyroid disorders.

Selenium: Selenium is essential for the proper functioning of the thyroid gland as it helps to convert T4 into T3, the more active thyroid hormone. Selenium also plays a role in protecting the thyroid gland from oxidative stress. Foods rich in selenium include Brazil nuts, seafood, and mushrooms.

Zinc: Zinc contributes to thyroid hormone metabolism and the conversion of T4 to T3. It is also important for the function of the hypothalamus, which signals the pituitary gland to release thyroid-stimulating hormone (TSH), which then stimulates the thyroid. Zinc can be found in meat, shellfish, nuts, and legumes.

Iron: Iron deficiency has been linked to decreased thyroid function and hypothyroidism. The thyroid needs iron to produce thyroid hormone, and iron deficiency can impair hormone production. Sources of iron include red meat, poultry, lentils, and fortified cereals.

Tyrosine: This amino acid is a building block for thyroid hormones. Tyrosine, combined with iodine, helps form T3 and T4. Foods high in protein, such as chicken, turkey, dairy products, and nuts, are good sources of tyrosine.

Dietary Patterns and Thyroid Health

Balanced Intake of Goitrogens: Goitrogens are substances in food that can interfere with thyroid function by inhibiting iodine uptake. Foods such as cruciferous vegetables (e.g., broccoli, cauliflower, cabbage, and Brussels sprouts) and soy products contain goitrogens. Although these foods are healthy, they should be consumed in moderation, particularly by those with existing thyroid issues, and it's beneficial to cook these vegetables to reduce their goitrogenic activity.

Gluten and Thyroid Autoimmunity: For individuals with Hashimoto's thyroiditis, a common thyroid disorder, gluten can sometimes exacerbate the condition. This is due to a potential molecular mimicry scenario where the immune system may mistake thyroid cells for gliadin (a component of gluten), leading to an immune attack on the thyroid.

Weight Management and Metabolic Impact: Since the thyroid regulates metabolic processes, maintaining a healthy weight can help manage thyroid disorders. A balanced diet that supports metabolic health can contribute to overall thyroid health.

Nutritional Therapy for Thyroid Health

Optimal Dietary Practices:

- Eating whole, unprocessed foods as much as possible.
- Ensuring a balanced intake of carbohydrates, proteins, and fats.
- Incorporating a variety of fruits and vegetables to provide essential vitamins and antioxidants that support the immune system and overall health.
- Staying hydrated, as water helps with metabolism and detoxification.

Supplementation: While food sources are the best way to get nutrients, sometimes supplementation may be necessary, especially in cases of nutrient deficiencies which can affect thyroid function. It is crucial to consult with a healthcare provider before starting any supplements, particularly because certain supplements can interact with thyroid medications.

ELIMINATION PROVOCATION DIET GUIDELINES

An Elimination Provocation Diet, often simply called an elimination diet, is a method used to identify foods that an individual may be sensitive to, which could potentially affect their health—including thyroid health. This approach involves removing specific foods or food groups from the diet for a period of time and then gradually reintroducing them to observe possible symptoms or reactions. This can be particularly useful for individuals dealing with thyroid issues, as dietary sensitivities can exacerbate symptoms or interfere with thyroid function.

Understanding the Elimination Diet
The premise behind an elimination diet is to pinpoint foods that trigger inflammation, immune responses, or hormonal imbalances which can negatively impact the thyroid. Common triggers might include gluten, dairy, soy, eggs, nuts, seeds, nightshades, and specific additives or preservatives.

Guidelines for Implementing Your Own Personal Elimination Provocation Diet
1. Planning and Preparation
- **Consult with a Professional:** Begin by consulting with a healthcare provider or a registered dietitian who is knowledgeable about thyroid health and elimination diets. They can offer guidance tailored to your specific health needs.
- **Choose What to Eliminate:** Typically, you start by eliminating common allergens and foods known to impact thyroid health negatively. For thyroid-specific concerns, it's common to eliminate gluten, dairy, soy, and processed sugars first.

2. Elimination Phase
- **Remove Selected Foods:** Completely eliminate the chosen foods from your diet. This phase usually lasts about 4-6 weeks. It's important to read labels and ask about ingredients when eating out to ensure you're not consuming the eliminated foods inadvertently.
- **Keep a Diary:** During this phase, keep a detailed food diary. Record everything you eat and note any changes in your symptoms. This can help identify correlations between symptoms and dietary intake.

3. Reintroduction Phase

- **Introduce Foods One at a Time:** After the elimination phase, reintroduce one food group at a time. Typically, you add a food back into your diet for a day and then return to the elimination diet for the next 2-3 days. During this period, observe and document any changes in symptoms.
- **Evaluate the Reaction:** If a food causes no reaction, it can be reincorporated into the diet. However, if symptoms reappear or worsen, it is likely a trigger and should be avoided.

4. Establishing a Long-Term Plan

- **Modify Your Diet:** Based on your findings, modify your long-term eating habits to exclude any foods that cause adverse reactions.
- **Periodic Reassessment:** Over time, it's possible that your tolerance to certain foods may change. It can be useful to retry eliminating and reintroducing foods annually or when symptoms change.

BREAKFAST RECIPES

1. Pear and Walnut Salad

Ingredients:

- 2 ripe pears, cored and sliced
- 1 cup walnuts, roughly chopped
- 4 cups mixed greens (spinach, arugula, and lettuce)
- 1/2 red onion, thinly sliced
- 1/4 cup crumbled feta cheese
- 2 tablespoons olive oil
- 1 tablespoon balsamic vinegar
- 1 teaspoon honey
- Salt and pepper, to taste

Instructions:

1. In a large salad bowl, combine the mixed greens, sliced pears, red onion, and walnuts.
2. In a small bowl, whisk together olive oil, balsamic vinegar, honey, salt, and pepper to create the dressing.
3. Drizzle the dressing over the salad and toss gently to combine.
4. Sprinkle crumbled feta cheese over the top just before serving.

Nutrition Info Per Serving:

- Calories: 270
- Fat: 21g
- Carbohydrates: 18g
- Protein: 5g
- Fiber: 4g

Serves: 4 Cooking Time: 10 minutes

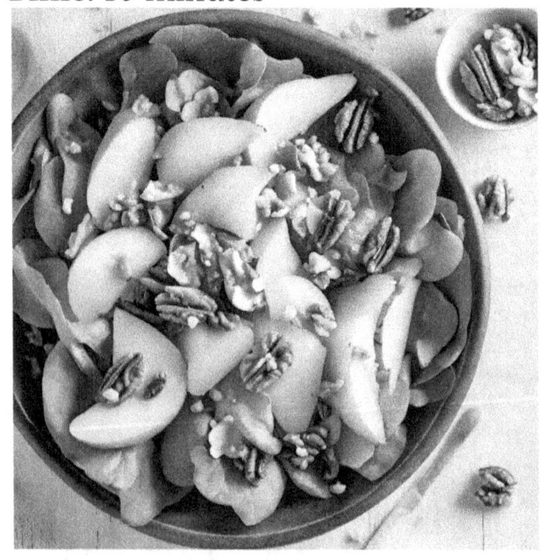

2. Ricotta and Berry Tarts

Ingredients:

- 4 whole grain tart shells, prebaked
- 1 cup ricotta cheese
- 2 tablespoons honey
- 1 teaspoon vanilla extract
- 1 cup mixed berries (raspberries, blueberries, blackberries)
- Mint leaves, for garnish

Instructions:

1. In a mixing bowl, combine ricotta cheese, honey, and vanilla extract. Mix until smooth.
2. Spoon the ricotta mixture into the prebaked tart shells.
3. Top each tart with a generous amount of mixed berries.
4. Garnish with mint leaves.
5. Serve immediately or chill in the refrigerator until ready to serve.

Nutrition Info Per Serving:

- Calories: 220
- Fat: 12g
- Carbohydrates: 20g
- Protein: 8g
- Fiber: 3g

Serves: 4 **Cooking Time:** 15 minutes

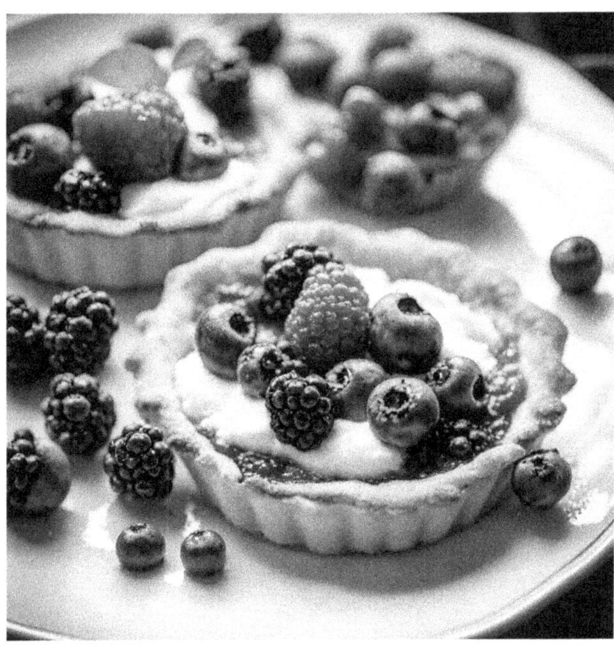

3. Melon and Prosciutto Plate

Ingredients:

- 1 medium cantaloupe, sliced into wedges
- 8 slices of prosciutto
- 1/4 cup balsamic glaze
- Fresh basil leaves, for garnish

Instructions:

1. Arrange cantaloupe wedges on a platter.
2. Carefully wrap each slice of prosciutto around a cantaloupe wedge.
3. Drizzle balsamic glaze over the wrapped cantaloupe.
4. Garnish with fresh basil leaves.
5. Serve immediately.

Nutrition Info Per Serving:

- Calories: 180
- Fat: 7g
- Carbohydrates: 21g
- Protein: 10g
- Fiber: 2g

Serves: 4 **Cooking Time:** 10 minutes

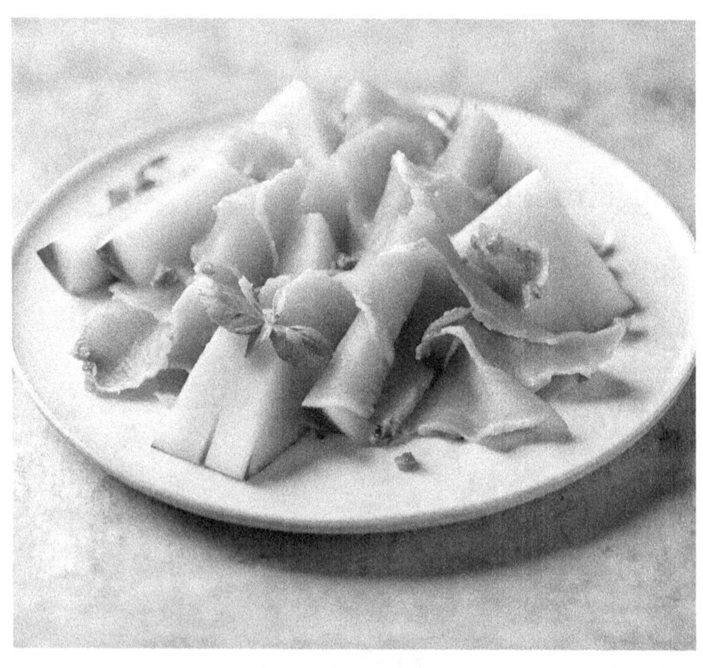

4. Cucumber and Herb Salad with Feta

Ingredients:

- 2 large cucumbers, peeled and thinly sliced
- 1/2 cup fresh parsley, chopped
- 1/4 cup fresh mint, chopped
- 1/4 cup fresh dill, chopped
- 1/2 red onion, thinly sliced
- 1 cup crumbled feta cheese
- 2 tablespoons olive oil
- Juice of 1 lemon
- Salt and pepper, to taste

Instructions:

1. In a large bowl, combine the cucumber slices, parsley, mint, dill, and red onion.
2. In a small bowl, whisk together the olive oil, lemon juice, salt, and pepper to make the dressing.
3. Pour the dressing over the salad and toss to coat evenly.
4. Sprinkle crumbled feta cheese over the top and gently mix.
5. Serve chilled or at room temperature.

Nutrition Info Per Serving:

- Calories: 180
- Fat: 14g
- Carbohydrates: 10g
- Protein: 6g
- Fiber: 2g

Serves: 4 **Cooking Time:** 15 minutes

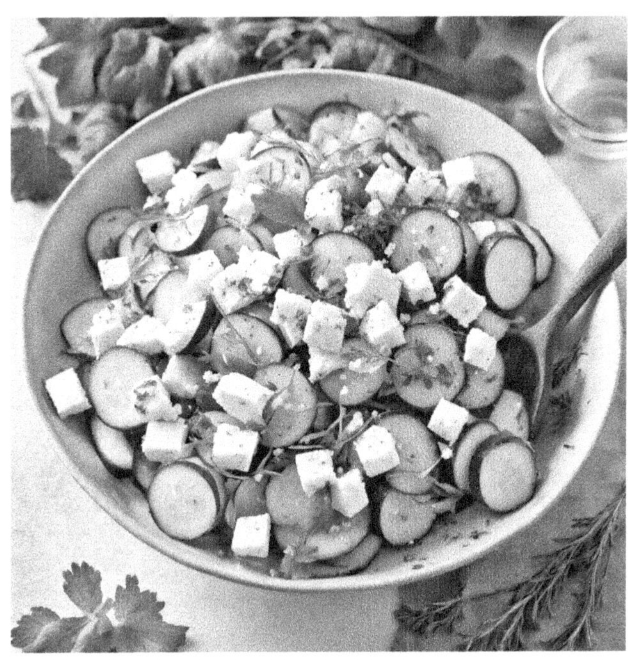

5. Nutty Yogurt Bowl

Ingredients:

- 2 cups plain Greek yogurt
- 1/4 cup honey
- 1/2 cup mixed nuts (almonds, walnuts, hazelnuts), chopped
- 1 banana, sliced
- 1/4 cup dried cranberries
- 1 teaspoon ground cinnamon

Instructions:

1. Divide the Greek yogurt into 4 bowls.
2. Drizzle honey evenly over each serving of yogurt.
3. Top with chopped nuts, banana slices, dried cranberries, and a sprinkle of cinnamon.
4. Serve immediately.

Nutrition Info Per Serving:

- Calories: 320
- Fat: 15g
- Carbohydrates: 36g
- Protein: 14g
- Fiber: 4g

Serves: 4 Cooking Time: 5 minutes

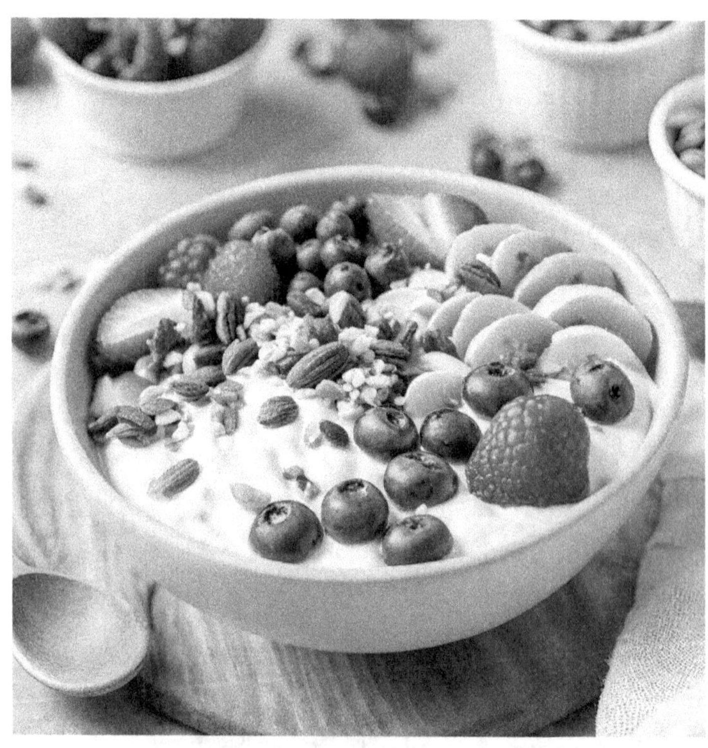

6. Breakfast Veggie Pockets

Ingredients:

- 4 whole wheat pita breads
- 1 cup cooked and drained spinach
- 1/2 cup cherry tomatoes, halved
- 1/4 cup sliced black olives
- 1/2 cup shredded mozzarella cheese
- 4 eggs, scrambled
- Salt and pepper, to taste
- Olive oil for brushing

Instructions:

1. Preheat your oven to 350°F (175°C).
2. Scramble the eggs in a skillet and season with salt and pepper.
3. Slice the pita breads in half to make pockets and brush the outside lightly with olive oil.
4. Stuff each pita pocket with an equal amount of scrambled eggs, spinach, tomatoes, black olives, and mozzarella cheese.
5. Place the stuffed pitas on a baking sheet and bake for 10 minutes, or until the pitas are crispy and the cheese is melted.
6. Serve warm.

Nutrition Info Per Serving:

- Calories: 300
- Fat: 15g
- Carbohydrates: 30g
- Protein: 16g
- Fiber: 5g

Serves: 4 **Cooking Time:** 20 minutes

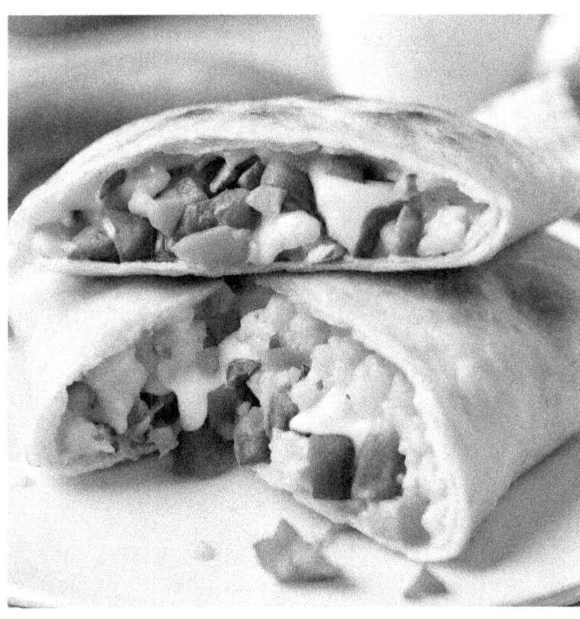

7. Baked Avocado Eggs

Ingredients:

- 4 avocados, halved and pitted
- 8 eggs
- Salt and pepper, to taste
- 1/4 cup chopped chives for garnish

Instructions:

1. Preheat your oven to 425°F (220°C).
2. Scoop out a bit of the avocado from the center to make room for the eggs.
3. Crack an egg into each avocado half, and season with salt and pepper.
4. Place the avocado halves in a baking dish and bake for 15 minutes, or until the eggs are cooked to your liking.
5. Garnish with chopped chives and serve immediately.

Nutrition Info Per Serving:

- Calories: 240
- Fat: 20g
- Carbohydrates: 9g
- Protein: 8g
- Fiber: 7g

Serves: 4 (2 halves each) **Cooking Time:** 20 minutes

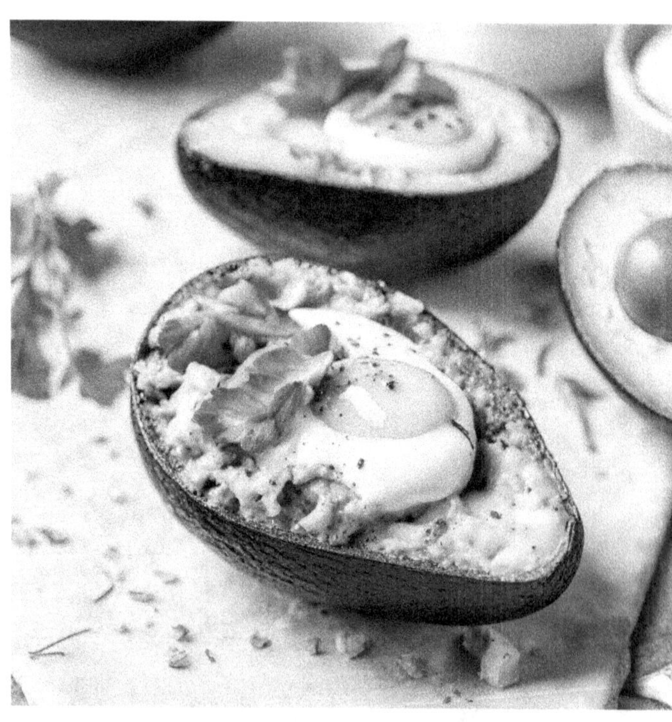

8. Greek Yogurt Parfait

Ingredients:

- 2 cups Greek yogurt, plain
- 1 cup granola
- 1 cup mixed berries (strawberries, blueberries, raspberries)
- 2 tablespoons honey
- 1/4 cup slivered almonds

Instructions:

1. In four serving glasses, layer 1/4 cup of Greek yogurt followed by a layer of granola and then a layer of mixed berries.
2. Repeat the layering process until all ingredients are used.
3. Drizzle honey over each parfait and sprinkle with slivered almonds.
4. Serve immediately or chill until ready to serve.

Nutrition Info Per Serving:

- Calories: 320
- Fat: 10g
- Carbohydrates: 44g
- Protein: 20g
- Fiber: 5g

Serves: 4 Cooking Time: 10 minutes

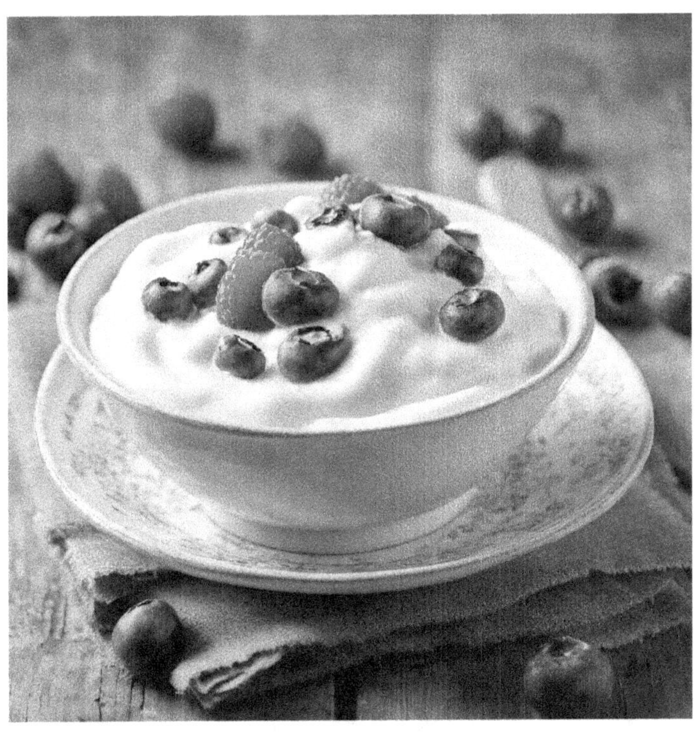

9. Turkey and Spinach Breakfast Hash

Ingredients:

- 1 pound ground turkey
- 2 cups spinach, chopped
- 1 large sweet potato, peeled and diced
- 1 medium onion, diced
- 2 cloves garlic, minced
- 2 tablespoons olive oil
- Salt and pepper, to taste

Instructions:

1. Heat olive oil in a large skillet over medium heat. Add diced sweet potato and onion, cooking until tender, about 10 minutes.
2. Add minced garlic and ground turkey, breaking up the meat as it cooks, until the turkey is browned and cooked through, about 8 minutes.
3. Stir in chopped spinach and cook until wilted, about 2 minutes.
4. Season with salt and pepper. Serve hot.

Nutrition Info Per Serving:

- Calories: 295
- Fat: 15g
- Carbohydrates: 18g
- Protein: 23g
- Fiber: 3g

Serves: 4 **Cooking Time:** 20 minutes

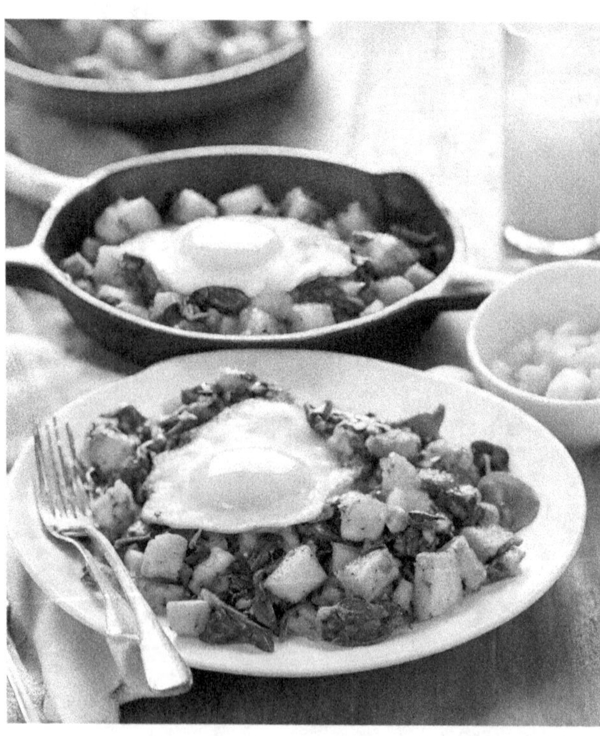

10. Sardine Salad

Ingredients:

- 2 cans sardines in olive oil, drained
- 1 small red onion, thinly sliced
- 1/2 cucumber, diced
- 1/2 cup cherry tomatoes, halved
- 1/4 cup chopped fresh parsley
- Juice of 1 lemon
- Salt and pepper, to taste

Instructions:

1. In a large bowl, combine sardines, red onion, cucumber, cherry tomatoes, and parsley.
2. Drizzle with lemon juice and season with salt and pepper to taste.
3. Toss gently to combine and serve chilled.

Nutrition Info Per Serving:

- Calories: 190
- Fat: 12g
- Carbohydrates: 6g
- Protein: 17g
- Fiber: 2g

Serves: 4 **Cooking Time:** 10 minutes

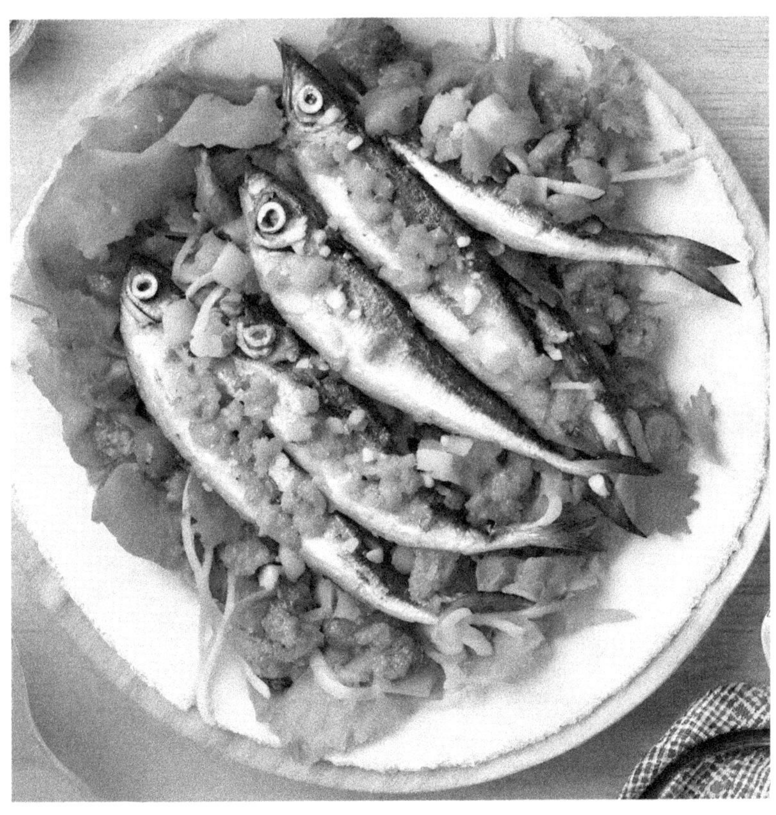

11. Tomato and Olive Tapenade on Toast

Ingredients:

- 4 slices whole grain bread
- 1 cup cherry tomatoes, quartered
- 1/2 cup black olives, pitted and chopped
- 1/4 cup fresh basil, chopped
- 2 tablespoons capers, drained
- 1 garlic clove, minced
- 3 tablespoons olive oil
- Salt and pepper, to taste

Instructions:

1. In a bowl, mix tomatoes, olives, basil, capers, minced garlic, and olive oil. Season with salt and pepper.
2. Toast the bread slices until golden.
3. Top each slice of toast with the tomato and olive tapenade.
4. Serve immediately.

Nutrition Info Per Serving:

- Calories: 220
- Fat: 14g
- Carbohydrates: 20g
- Protein: 4g
- Fiber: 3g

Serves: 4 **Cooking Time:** 15 minutes

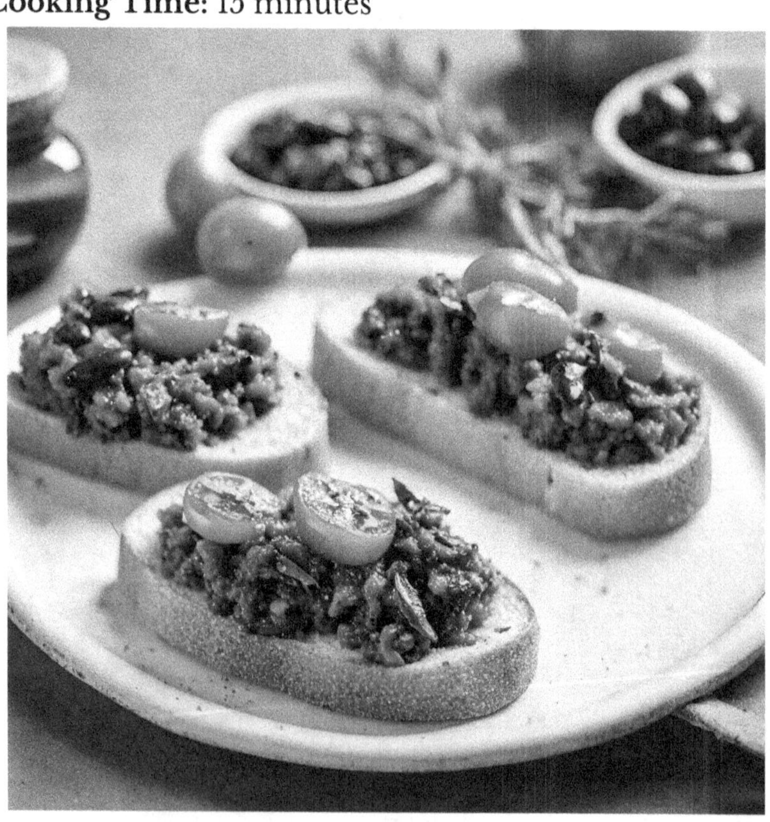

12. Smoked Turkey and Avocado Sandwich

Ingredients:

- 8 slices whole grain bread
- 8 ounces smoked turkey, sliced
- 1 avocado, sliced
- 1 tomato, sliced
- 4 lettuce leaves
- 2 tablespoons mayonnaise
- 1 tablespoon mustard

Instructions:

1. Spread mayonnaise and mustard on 4 slices of bread.
2. Layer each with turkey, avocado slices, tomato slices, and a lettuce leaf.
3. Top with the remaining bread slices.
4. Cut sandwiches in half and serve.

Nutrition Info Per Serving:

- Calories: 350
- Fat: 18g
- Carbohydrates: 33g
- Protein: 20g
- Fiber: 6g

Serves: 4 **Cooking Time:** 10 minutes

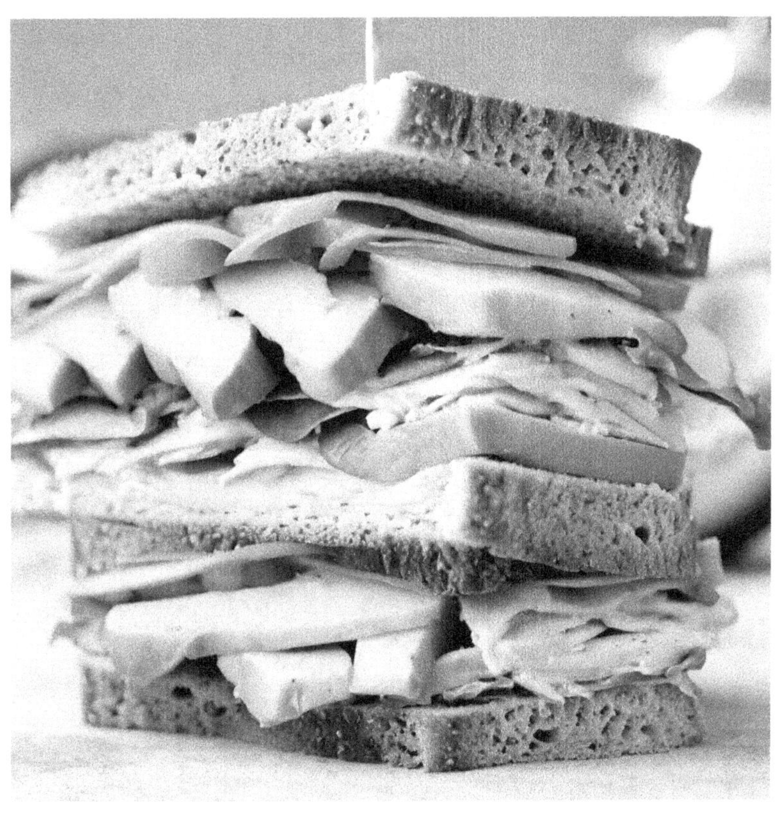

13. Cottage Cheese and Pineapple Toast

Ingredients:

- 4 slices of whole grain bread
- 1 cup cottage cheese
- 1 cup chopped pineapple
- 1 tablespoon honey
- 1 teaspoon ground cinnamon

Instructions:

1. Toast the bread slices until crisp.
2. Spread each slice evenly with cottage cheese.
3. Top with chopped pineapple, drizzle with honey, and sprinkle cinnamon over each.
4. Serve immediately.

Nutrition Info Per Serving:

- Calories: 210
- Fat: 3g
- Carbohydrates: 32g
- Protein: 12g
- Fiber: 4g

Serves: 4 **Cooking Time:** 10 minutes

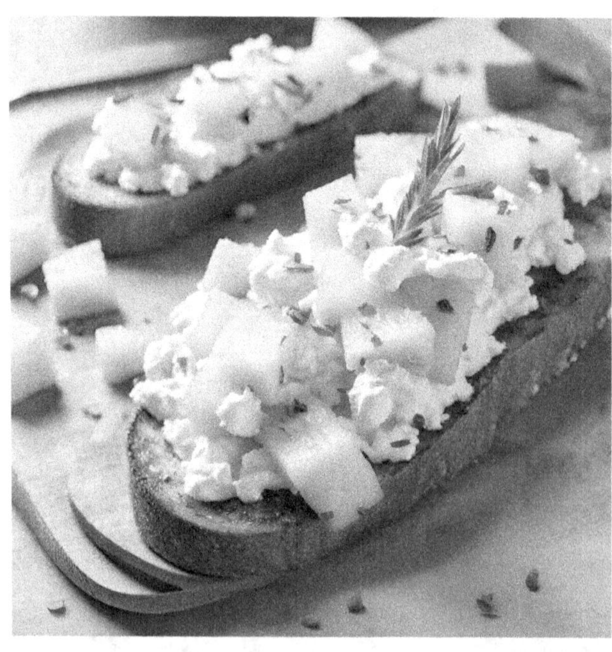

14. Almond Butter and Banana Sandwich

Ingredients:

- 8 slices whole grain bread
- 1/2 cup almond butter
- 2 bananas, sliced
- 1 teaspoon honey (optional)

Instructions:

1. Spread almond butter evenly on 4 slices of bread.
2. Arrange banana slices over the almond butter and drizzle with honey if using.
3. Top with the remaining bread slices.
4. Serve as is or lightly toasted.

Nutrition Info Per Serving:

- Calories: 350
- Fat: 18g
- Carbohydrates: 40g
- Protein: 10g
- Fiber: 7g

Serves: 4 **Cooking Time:** 5 minutes

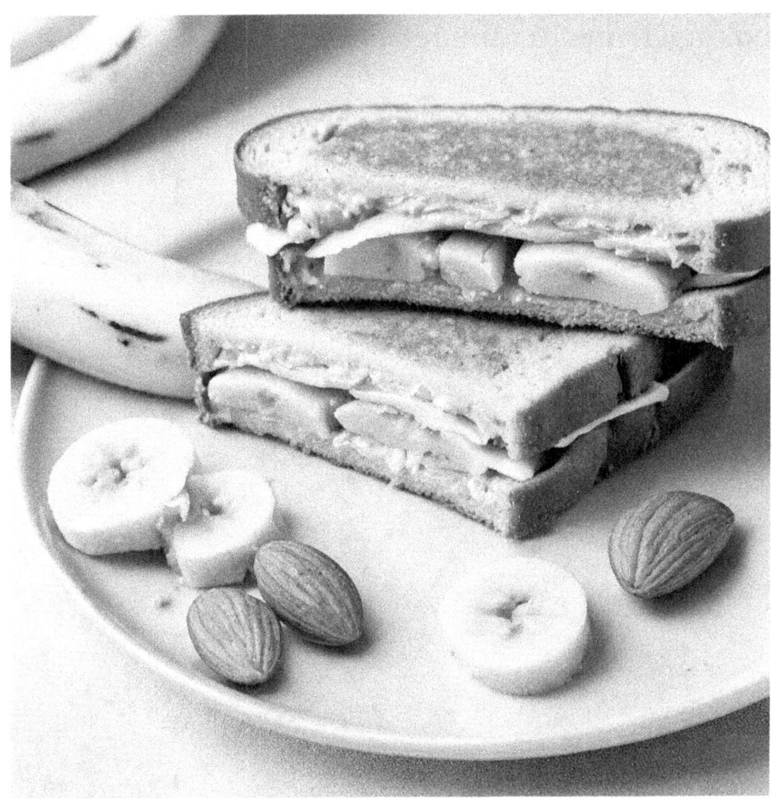

15. Avocado and Radish Toast

Ingredients:

- 4 slices of whole grain bread
- 2 avocados, mashed
- 8 radishes, thinly sliced
- 1/4 cup fresh cilantro, chopped
- Juice of 1 lime
- Salt and pepper, to taste

Instructions:

1. Toast the bread slices.
2. Spread mashed avocado on each slice.
3. Top with sliced radishes and sprinkle with chopped cilantro.
4. Drizzle lime juice over the top and season with salt and pepper.
5. Serve immediately.

Nutrition Info Per Serving:

- Calories: 250
- Fat: 15g
- Carbohydrates: 27g
- Protein: 6g
- Fiber: 9g

Serves: 4 Cooking Time: 10 minutes

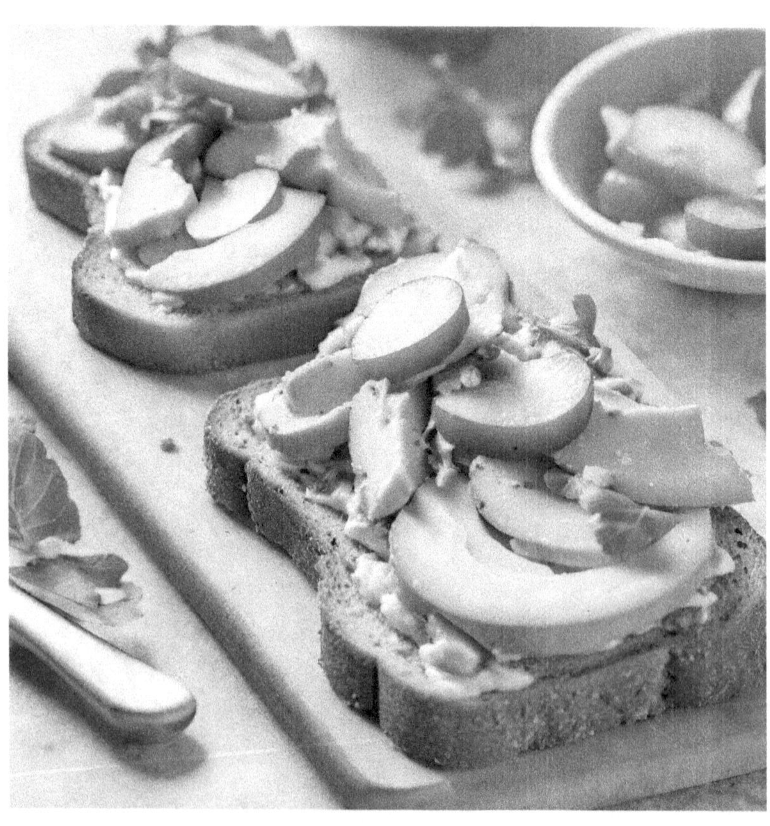

16. Creamy Millet Porridge

Ingredients:

- 1 cup millet
- 3 cups water
- 1 cup almond milk
- 2 tablespoons honey
- 1/2 teaspoon cinnamon
- 1/4 cup raisins
- 1/4 cup chopped walnuts

Instructions:

1. Rinse millet thoroughly in cold water.
2. In a medium saucepan, bring 3 cups of water to a boil. Add millet and reduce heat to a simmer. Cover and cook for 15 minutes until tender.
3. Stir in almond milk, honey, and cinnamon, and continue to cook for another 5 minutes until creamy.
4. Mix in raisins and walnuts before serving.

Nutrition Info Per Serving:

- Calories: 260
- Fat: 5g
- Carbohydrates: 47g
- Protein: 6g
- Fiber: 4g

Serves: 4 **Cooking Time:** 20 minutes

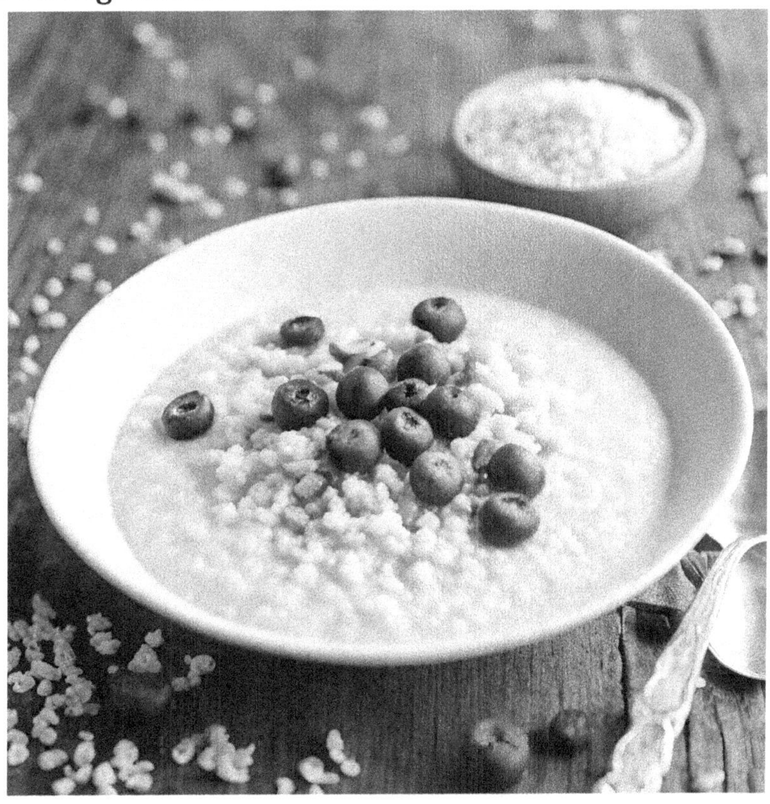

17. Warm Buckwheat Bowl

Ingredients:

- 1 cup buckwheat groats
- 3 cups water
- 1 apple, diced
- 1/4 teaspoon ground nutmeg
- 1/4 teaspoon ground ginger
- 1/4 cup dried cranberries
- 1/4 cup sliced almonds

Instructions:

1. Rinse buckwheat groats under cold water until water runs clear.
2. In a pot, bring 3 cups of water to a boil. Add buckwheat, reduce heat to low, cover, and simmer for 10 minutes.
3. Add diced apple, nutmeg, and ginger to the pot. Cook for another 5 minutes until the apple is soft.
4. Stir in dried cranberries and cook for an additional 5 minutes.
5. Serve hot, garnished with sliced almonds.

Nutrition Info Per Serving:

- Calories: 210
- Fat: 3g
- Carbohydrates: 40g
- Protein: 6g
- Fiber: 5g

Serves: 4 **Cooking Time:** 20 minutes

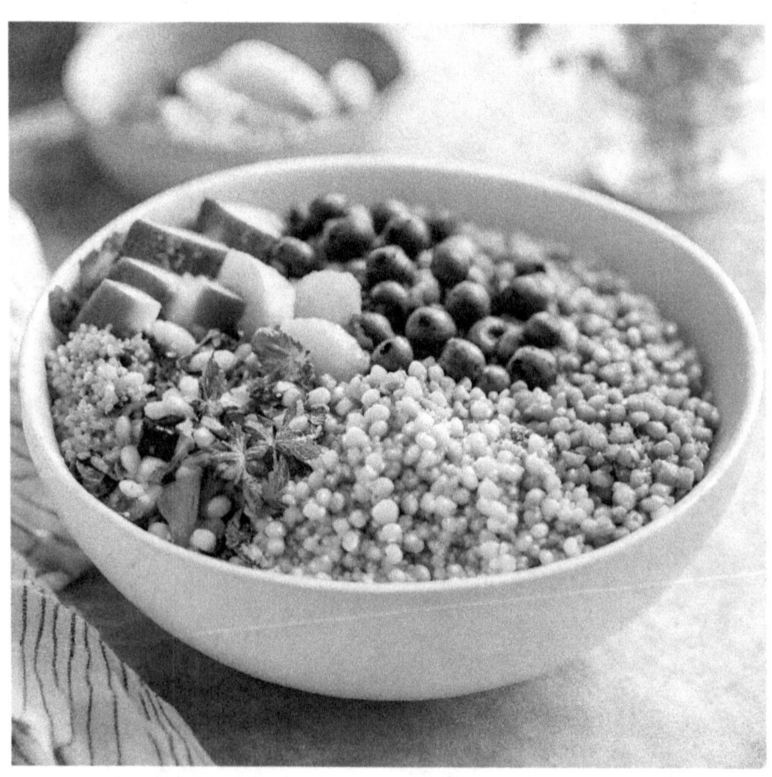

18. Quinoa Porridge with Almonds

Ingredients:

- 1 cup quinoa
- 2 cups water
- 1 cup unsweetened almond milk
- 1/4 cup sliced almonds
- 2 tablespoons maple syrup
- 1/2 teaspoon vanilla extract
- Pinch of salt

Instructions:

1. Rinse quinoa in cold water.
2. In a saucepan, combine quinoa and water. Bring to a boil, then reduce heat and simmer covered for 15 minutes.
3. Add almond milk, maple syrup, vanilla extract, and a pinch of salt. Stir and cook for another 5 minutes until thick and creamy.
4. Serve hot, topped with sliced almonds.

Nutrition Info Per Serving:

- Calories: 280
- Fat: 8g
- Carbohydrates: 44g
- Protein: 8g
- Fiber: 4g

Serves: 4 **Cooking Time:** 20 minutes

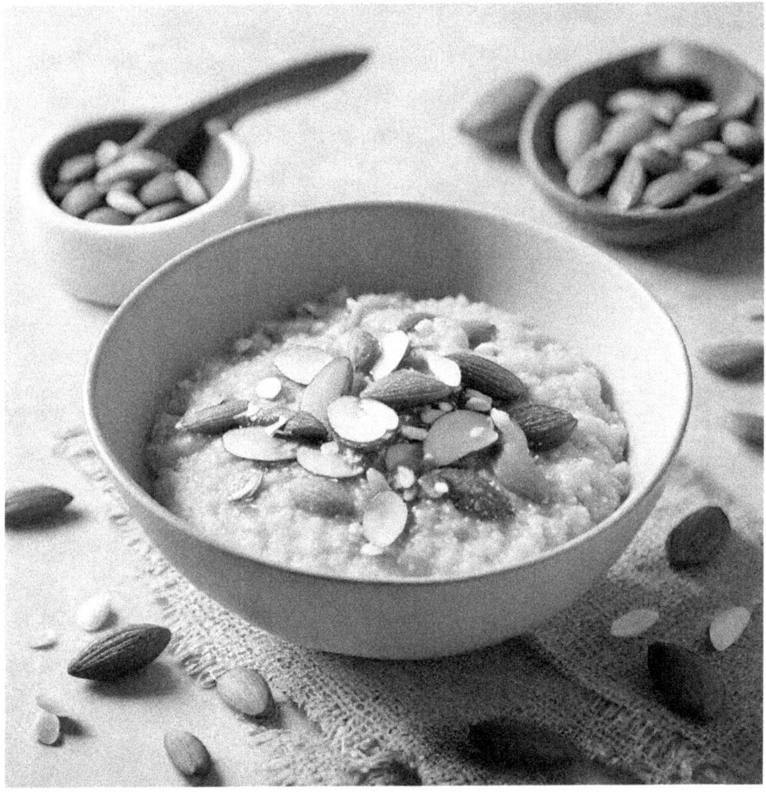

19. Chia and Lemon Pancakes

Ingredients:

- 1 cup all-purpose flour
- 1/4 cup chia seeds
- 1 tablespoon baking powder
- 1/4 teaspoon salt
- 1 cup milk
- 1 egg
- 2 tablespoons vegetable oil
- Zest of 1 lemon
- Juice of 1 lemon
- 2 tablespoons honey

Instructions:

1. In a bowl, combine flour, chia seeds, baking powder, and salt.
2. In another bowl, whisk together milk, egg, vegetable oil, lemon zest, and lemon juice.
3. Mix the wet ingredients into the dry ingredients until just combined. Let sit for 5 minutes.
4. Heat a non-stick skillet over medium heat. Pour 1/4 cup of batter for each pancake. Cook until bubbles form on the surface, then flip and cook until golden brown.
5. Serve hot with honey drizzled on top.

Nutrition Info Per Serving:

- Calories: 270
- Fat: 10g
- Carbohydrates: 39g
- Protein: 7g
- Fiber: 5g

Serves: 4 Cooking Time: 20 minutes

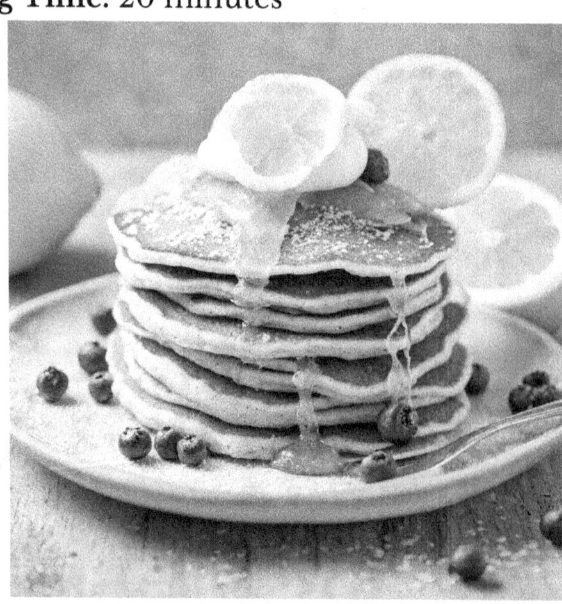

20. Buckwheat Blueberry Pancakes

Ingredients:
- 1 cup buckwheat flour
- 1 tablespoon sugar
- 1 teaspoon baking powder
- 1/2 teaspoon baking soda
- 1/4 teaspoon salt
- 1 cup buttermilk
- 1 egg
- 2 tablespoons melted butter
- 1 cup blueberries

Instructions:
1. In a large bowl, mix together buckwheat flour, sugar, baking powder, baking soda, and salt.
2. In another bowl, beat together buttermilk, egg, and melted butter.
3. Stir the wet ingredients into the dry ingredients until just combined. Fold in blueberries.
4. Heat a non-stick skillet over medium heat. Pour batter to form pancakes and cook until bubbles appear, then flip and cook until done.
5. Serve pancakes warm.

Nutrition Info Per Serving:
- Calories: 280
- Fat: 9g
- Carbohydrates: 42g
- Protein: 8g
- Fiber: 5g

Serves: 4 **Cooking Time:** 20 minutes

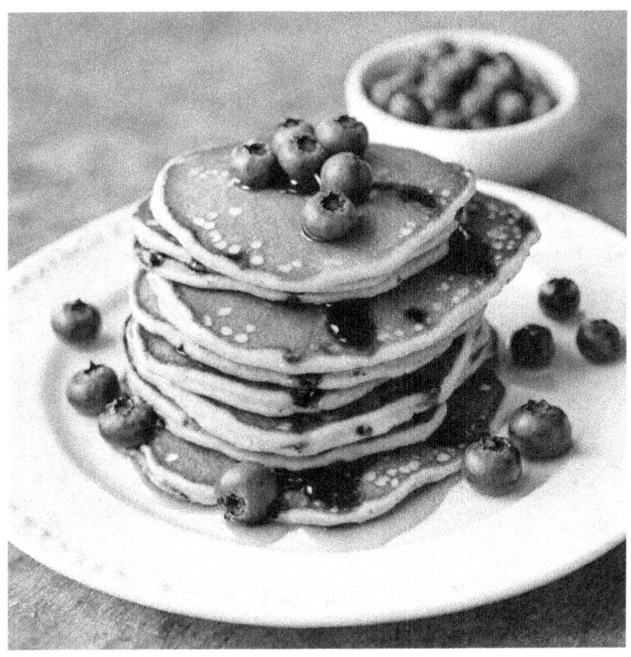

21. Banana Oat Pancakes
Ingredients:
- 1 cup rolled oats
- 1 banana, mashed
- 3/4 cup milk
- 1 egg
- 1 tablespoon honey
- 1/2 teaspoon baking powder
- 1/4 teaspoon salt
- Butter or oil for cooking

Instructions:
1. In a blender, combine oats, mashed banana, milk, egg, honey, baking powder, and salt. Blend until smooth.
2. Heat a lightly oiled griddle or frying pan over medium-high heat. Pour or scoop the batter onto the griddle, using approximately 1/4 cup for each pancake.
3. Cook until pancake is golden brown on both sides and serve hot.

Nutrition Info Per Serving:
- Calories: 220
- Fat: 5g
- Carbohydrates: 38g
- Protein: 7g
- Fiber: 4g

Serves: 4 **Cooking Time:** 15 minutes

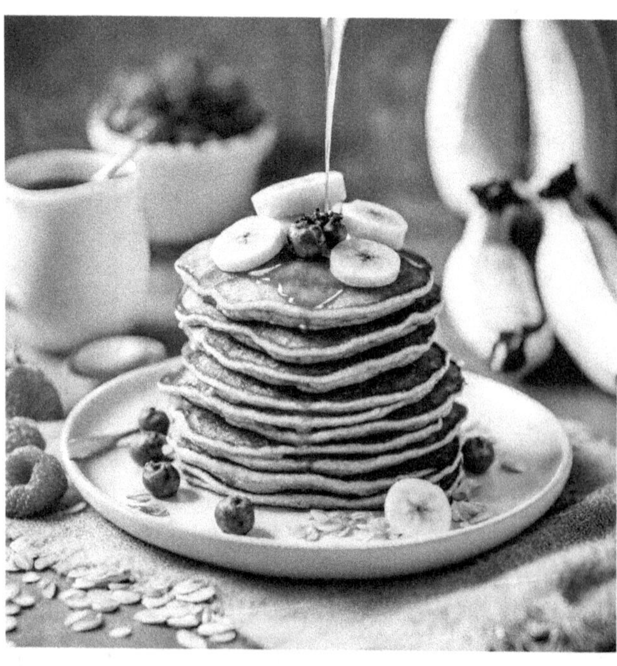

22. Coconut Flour Waffles

Ingredients:

- 1/2 cup coconut flour
- 1 teaspoon baking powder
- 1/4 teaspoon salt
- 4 eggs
- 1/4 cup coconut oil, melted
- 1/2 cup almond milk
- 2 tablespoons honey
- 1 teaspoon vanilla extract

Instructions:

1. In a bowl, mix coconut flour, baking powder, and salt.
2. In another bowl, whisk eggs, melted coconut oil, almond milk, honey, and vanilla extract.
3. Combine the wet and dry ingredients and mix until smooth.
4. Preheat a waffle iron and grease it lightly. Pour enough batter to cover the waffle iron grid. Close and cook until the waffle is golden and crisp.
5. Serve hot with your choice of toppings.

Nutrition Info Per Serving:

- Calories: 300
- Fat: 20g
- Carbohydrates: 20g
- Protein: 9g
- Fiber: 5g

Serves: 4 **Cooking Time:** 15 minutes

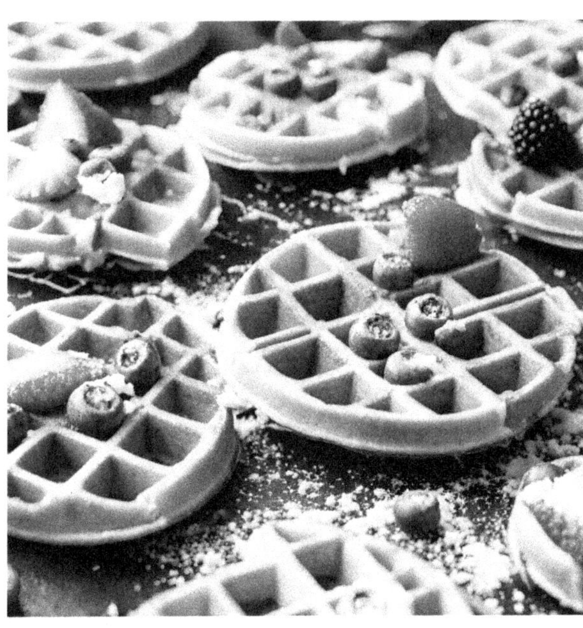

23. Almond Flour Pancakes

Ingredients:

- 1 cup almond flour
- 2 eggs
- 1/3 cup water
- 1 tablespoon maple syrup
- 1 teaspoon baking powder
- 1/4 teaspoon salt
- 1/2 teaspoon vanilla extract
- Butter or coconut oil, for cooking

Instructions:

1. In a bowl, mix almond flour, baking powder, and salt.
2. In another bowl, whisk eggs, water, maple syrup, and vanilla extract.
3. Combine wet and dry ingredients until a smooth batter forms.
4. Heat a non-stick skillet over medium heat and grease with butter or coconut oil.
5. Pour 1/4 cup of batter for each pancake. Cook until bubbles form on the surface, then flip and cook until golden brown on the other side.
6. Serve hot with additional maple syrup if desired.

Nutrition Info Per Serving:

- Calories: 265
- Fat: 21g
- Carbohydrates: 12g
- Protein: 10g
- Fiber: 3g

Serves: 4 **Cooking Time:** 15 minutes

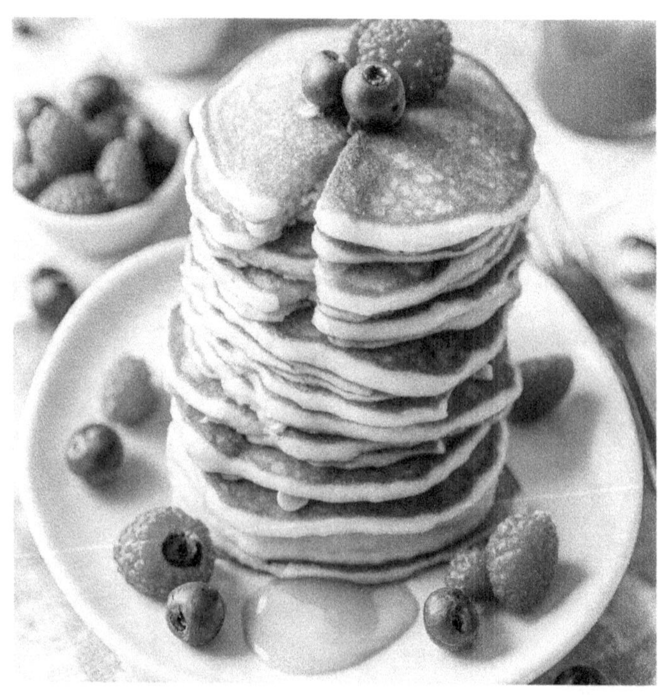

24. Sunny-Side Hemp Seeds

Ingredients:

- 4 large eggs
- 2 tablespoons hemp seeds
- 1 tablespoon olive oil
- Salt and pepper, to taste

Instructions:

1. Heat olive oil in a skillet over medium heat.
2. Crack eggs into the skillet, keeping the yolks intact.
3. Sprinkle hemp seeds over the eggs.
4. Season with salt and pepper.
5. Cook until the whites are fully set but the yolks are still runny, about 4-5 minutes.
6. Serve immediately.

Nutrition Info Per Serving:

- Calories: 155
- Fat: 12g
- Carbohydrates: 1g
- Protein: 11g
- Fiber: 0g

Serves: 4 **Cooking Time:** 10 minutes

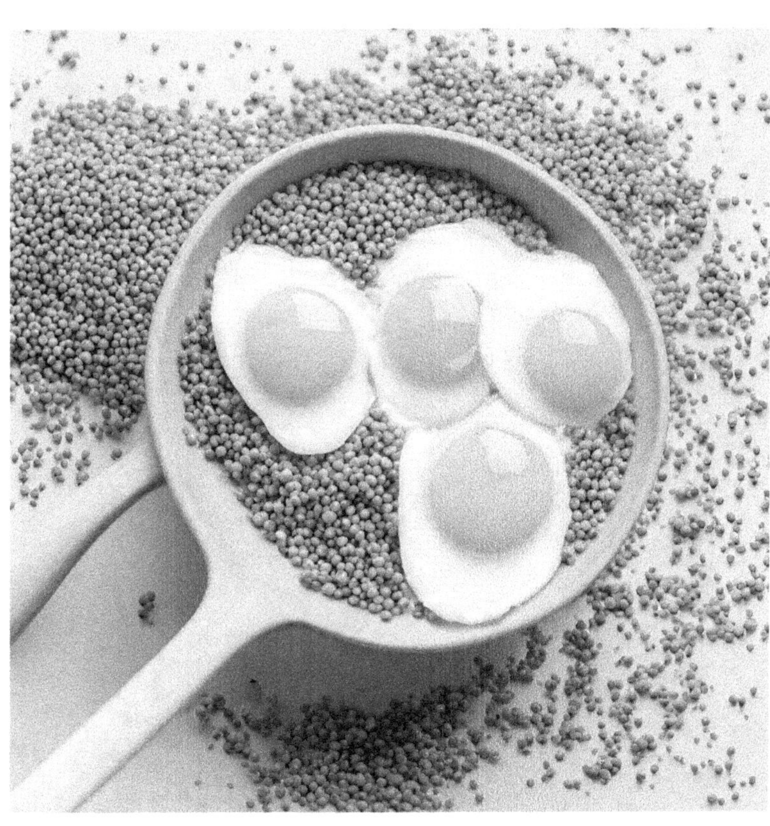

25. Tomato Avocado Egg Muffins
Ingredients:
- 6 eggs
- 1 avocado, diced
- 1/2 cup diced tomatoes
- 1/4 cup chopped onions
- 1/4 teaspoon salt
- 1/4 teaspoon pepper
- Cooking spray or oil for greasing

Instructions:
1. Preheat the oven to 350°F (175°C).
2. Grease a muffin tin with cooking spray or oil.
3. In a bowl, whisk together eggs, salt, and pepper.
4. Stir in diced avocado, tomatoes, and onions.
5. Pour the mixture into the muffin tins, filling each about three-quarters full.
6. Bake for 15-20 minutes, or until the eggs are set.
7. Let cool for a few minutes before removing from the tin and serving.

Nutrition Info Per Serving:
- Calories: 150
- Fat: 11g
- Carbohydrates: 5g
- Protein: 9g
- Fiber: 2g

Serves: 6 Cooking Time: 25 minutes

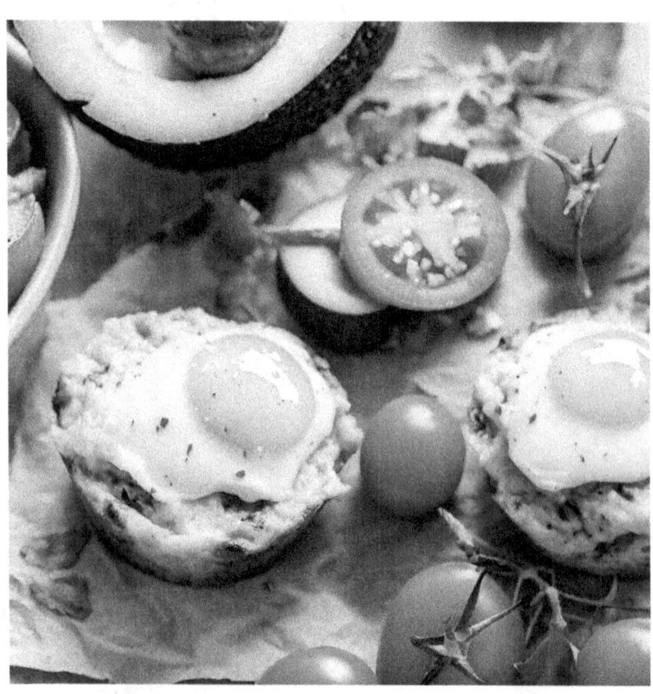

26. Iodine-Rich Seaweed Smoothie

Ingredients:

- 1 cup fresh spinach
- 1/2 cup dried seaweed (e.g., wakame), soaked and drained
- 1 banana
- 1/2 cup Greek yogurt
- 1 cup almond milk
- 1 tablespoon honey
- Ice cubes (optional)

Instructions:

1. Combine all ingredients in a blender.
2. Blend on high until smooth.
3. Serve immediately, adding ice cubes for a colder smoothie if desired.

Nutrition Info Per Serving:

- Calories: 180
- Fat: 3g
- Carbohydrates: 33g
- Protein: 8g
- Fiber: 4g

Serves: 2 **Cooking Time:** 5 minutes

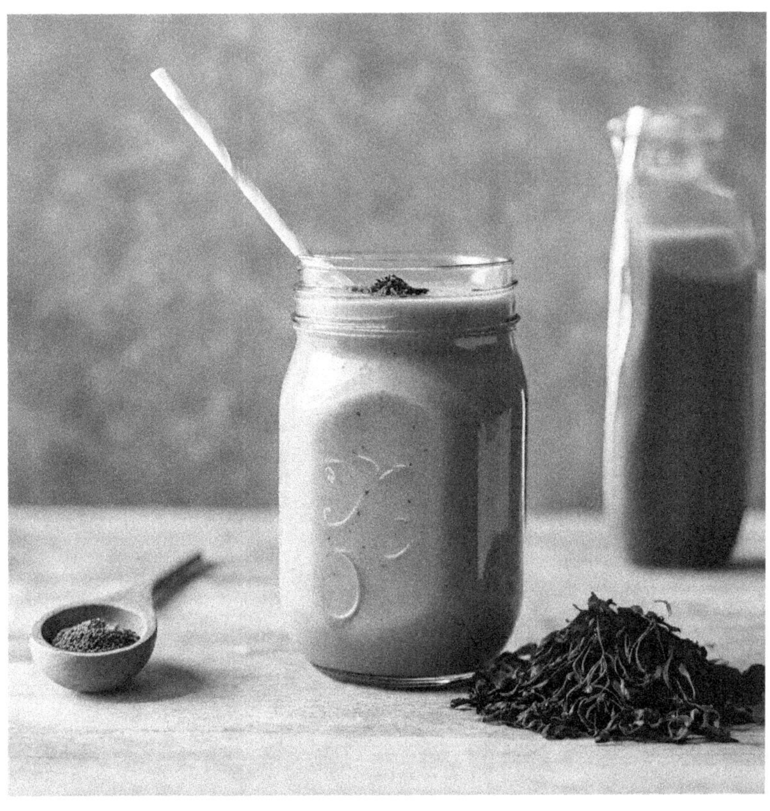

27. Berry Selenium Boost Smoothie
Ingredients:
- 1 cup frozen mixed berries (strawberries, blueberries, raspberries)
- 1 banana
- 1/2 cup Greek yogurt
- 1/4 cup Brazil nuts
- 1 cup orange juice
- 1 tablespoon flaxseeds

Instructions:
1. Combine all ingredients in a blender.
2. Blend until smooth.
3. Serve chilled.

Nutrition Info Per Serving:
- Calories: 285
- Fat: 12g
- Carbohydrates: 40g
- Protein: 10g
- Fiber: 5g

Serves: 2 Cooking Time: 5 minutes

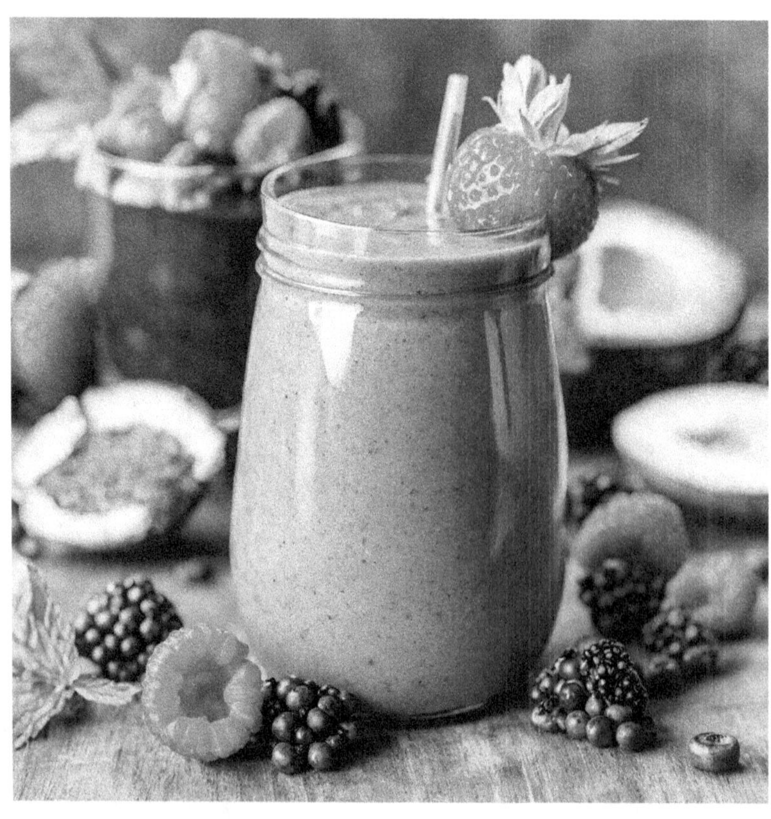

Soup & Salad Recipes

1. Carrot Ginger Soup

Ingredients:

- 2 tablespoons olive oil
- 1 onion, chopped
- 2 cloves garlic, minced
- 2 tablespoons fresh ginger, minced
- 1 pound carrots, peeled and diced
- 4 cups vegetable broth
- Salt and pepper, to taste
- 1/2 cup coconut milk (optional, for creaminess)

Instructions:

1. Heat olive oil in a large pot over medium heat. Add chopped onion and sauté until translucent, about 5 minutes.
2. Add minced garlic and ginger, cook for another 2 minutes until fragrant.
3. Add diced carrots and vegetable broth. Bring to a boil, then reduce heat and simmer until carrots are tender, about 20 minutes.
4. Puree the soup using an immersion blender or in batches with a regular blender until smooth.
5. Stir in coconut milk if using, season with salt and pepper, and heat through.
6. Serve hot.

Nutrition Info Per Serving:

- Calories: 180
- Fat: 7g
- Carbohydrates: 27g
- Protein: 3g
- Fiber: 6g

Serves: 4 **Cooking Time:** 30 minutes

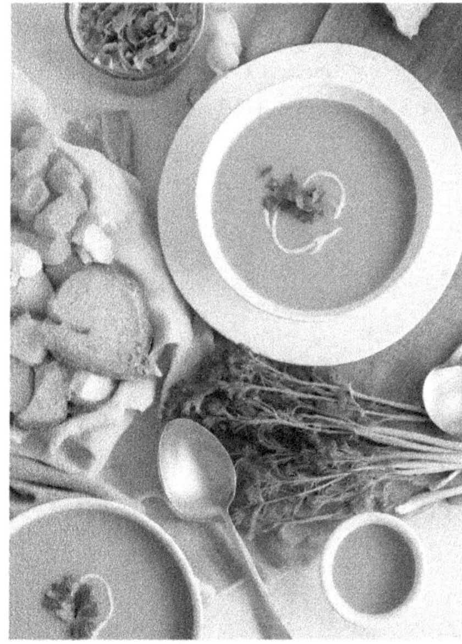

2. Tomato Basil Soup

Ingredients:

- 2 tablespoons olive oil
- 1 onion, diced
- 3 cloves garlic, minced
- 2 cans (28 ounces each) crushed tomatoes
- 4 cups vegetable broth
- 1/2 cup fresh basil, chopped
- Salt and pepper, to taste
- 1/2 cup heavy cream (optional)

Instructions:

1. In a large pot, heat olive oil over medium heat. Add onion and garlic, sauté until softened, about 5 minutes.
2. Stir in crushed tomatoes and vegetable broth. Bring to a simmer.
3. Add chopped basil, salt, and pepper. Continue to simmer for 15 minutes.
4. Blend the soup until smooth with an immersion blender or in a regular blender in batches.
5. Return the soup to the pot, stir in heavy cream if using, and heat through.
6. Serve hot garnished with extra basil.

Nutrition Info Per Serving:

- Calories: 220
- Fat: 14g
- Carbohydrates: 22g
- Protein: 4g
- Fiber: 4g

Serves: 4 Cooking Time: 25 minutes

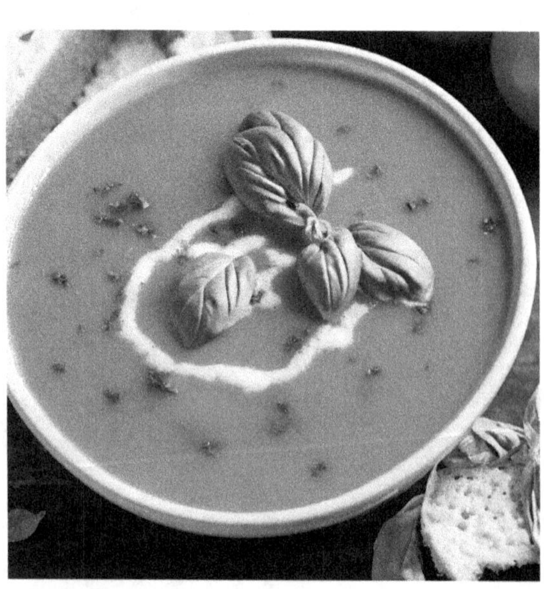

3. Kale and Quinoa Salad

Ingredients:

- 2 cups cooked quinoa
- 4 cups chopped kale, stems removed
- 1/2 cup dried cranberries
- 1/2 cup slivered almonds, toasted
- 1/4 cup feta cheese, crumbled
- For the dressing:
  - 1/4 cup olive oil
  - 2 tablespoons apple cider vinegar
  - 1 tablespoon honey
  - 1 teaspoon Dijon mustard
  - Salt and pepper, to taste

Instructions:

1. In a large salad bowl, combine cooked quinoa, chopped kale, dried cranberries, and slivered almonds.
2. In a small bowl, whisk together olive oil, apple cider vinegar, honey, Dijon mustard, salt, and pepper to create the dressing.
3. Drizzle the dressing over the salad and toss to coat thoroughly.
4. Sprinkle crumbled feta cheese over the salad before serving.

Nutrition Info Per Serving:

- Calories: 315
- Fat: 18g
- Carbohydrates: 34g
- Protein: 9g
- Fiber: 6g

Serves: 4 **Cooking Time:** 15 minutes (plus time to cook quinoa)

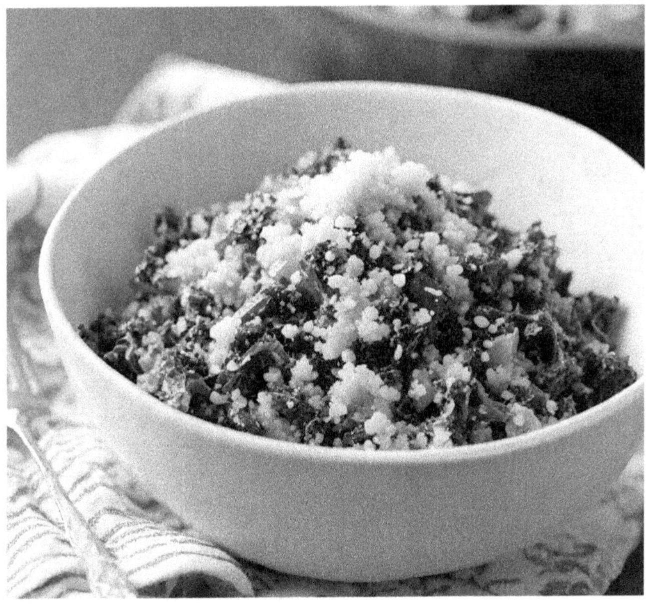

4. Spinach and Avocado Salad
Ingredients:

- 4 cups baby spinach
- 2 ripe avocados, diced
- 1/2 cup cherry tomatoes, halved
- 1/4 cup pine nuts, toasted
- 2 tablespoons olive oil
- 1 tablespoon balsamic vinegar
- Salt and pepper, to taste

Instructions:

1. In a large salad bowl, combine baby spinach, diced avocados, cherry tomatoes, and toasted pine nuts.
2. In a small bowl, whisk together olive oil and balsamic vinegar, season with salt and pepper.
3. Drizzle the dressing over the salad and toss gently to mix.
4. Serve immediately to maintain the freshness of the ingredients.

Nutrition Info Per Serving:

- Calories: 290
- Fat: 25g
- Carbohydrates: 17g
- Protein: 4g
- Fiber: 7g

Serves: 4 **Cooking Time:** 10 minutes

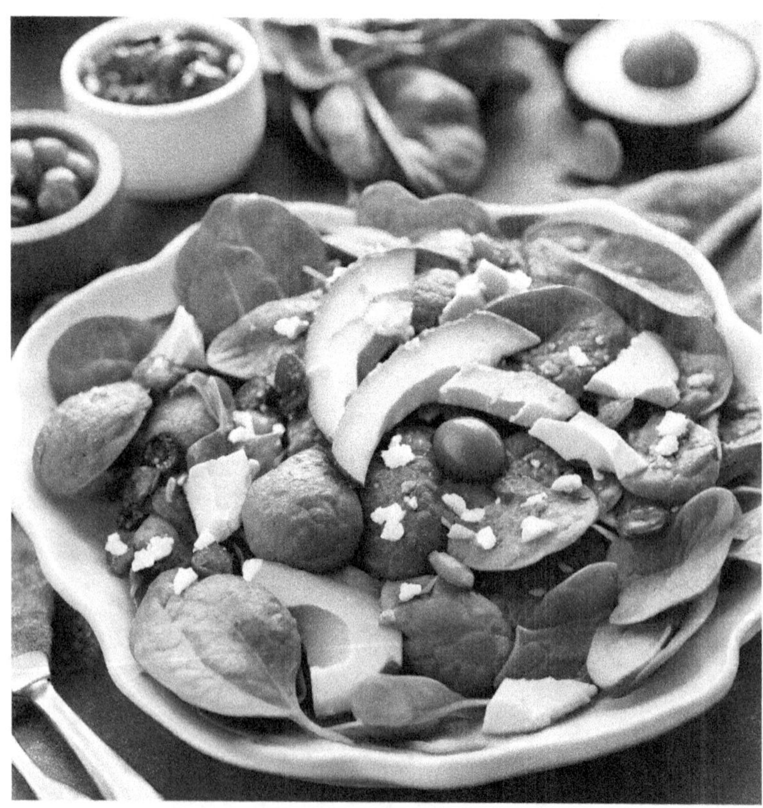

5. Spinach and White Bean Soup

Ingredients:

- 2 tablespoons olive oil
- 1 onion, diced
- 2 garlic cloves, minced
- 4 cups vegetable broth
- 1 can (15 oz) white beans, drained and rinsed
- 4 cups fresh spinach
- 1 teaspoon dried thyme
- Salt and pepper, to taste
- Grated Parmesan cheese (optional)

Instructions:

1. Heat olive oil in a large pot over medium heat. Add onion and garlic, and sauté until softened, about 5 minutes.
2. Add vegetable broth, white beans, and thyme. Bring to a boil, then reduce heat and simmer for 15 minutes.
3. Stir in spinach and cook until wilted, about 2 minutes.
4. Season with salt and pepper. Serve hot, garnished with Parmesan cheese if desired.

Nutrition Info Per Serving:

- Calories: 190
- Fat: 5g
- Carbohydrates: 27g
- Protein: 11g
- Fiber: 6g

Serves: 4 **Cooking Time:** 25 minutes

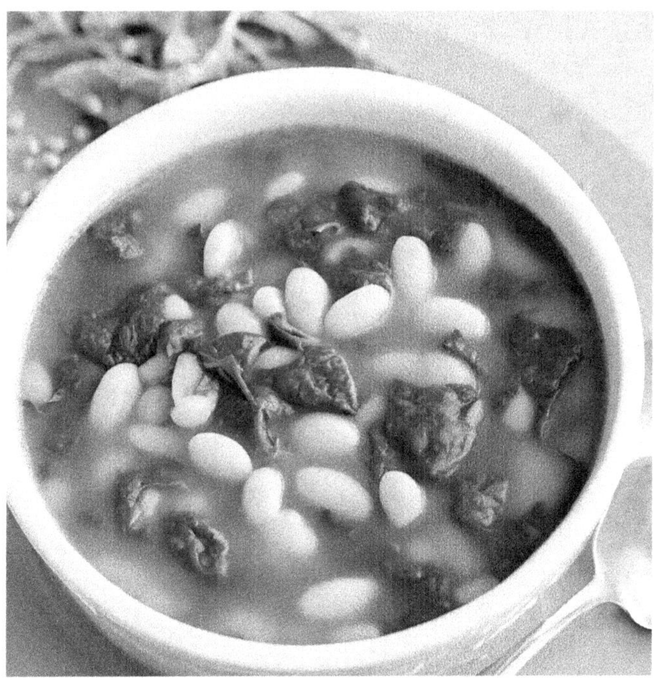

6. Roasted Red Pepper Soup

Ingredients:

- 2 tablespoons olive oil
- 1 onion, chopped
- 2 cloves garlic, minced
- 4 roasted red peppers, peeled and chopped
- 4 cups vegetable broth
- 1/2 teaspoon smoked paprika
- Salt and pepper, to taste
- 1/2 cup heavy cream (optional)

Instructions:

1. In a large pot, heat olive oil over medium heat. Add onion and garlic, and sauté until translucent, about 5 minutes.
2. Add roasted red peppers and paprika, cooking for another 2 minutes.
3. Pour in vegetable broth and bring to a boil. Reduce heat and simmer for 20 minutes.
4. Puree the soup in batches in a blender or use an immersion blender until smooth.
5. Stir in heavy cream if using, season with salt and pepper, and heat through.
6. Serve hot.

Nutrition Info Per Serving:

- Calories: 180
- Fat: 12g (if adding cream)
- Carbohydrates: 15g
- Protein: 3g
- Fiber: 2g

Serves: 4 **Cooking Time:** 30 minutes

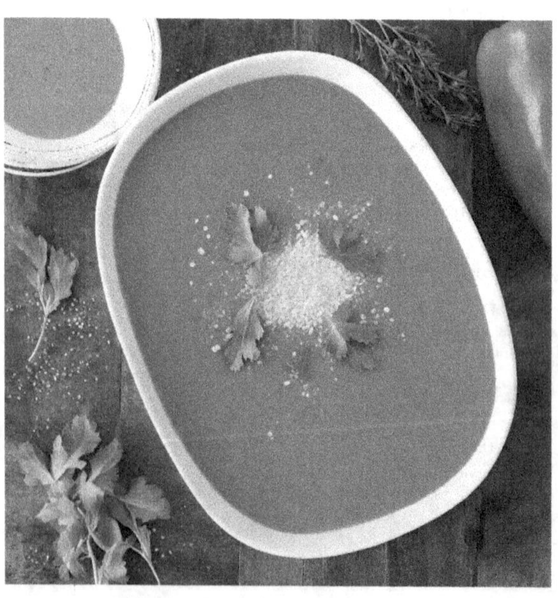

7. Butternut Squash Soup

Ingredients:

- 2 tablespoons olive oil
- 1 onion, diced
- 2 garlic cloves, minced
- 1 medium butternut squash, peeled, seeded, and cubed
- 4 cups vegetable broth
- 1 teaspoon cinnamon
- Salt and pepper, to taste

Instructions:

1. In a large pot, heat olive oil over medium heat. Add onion and garlic, sauté until soft.
2. Add squash, broth, and cinnamon. Bring to a boil, then reduce heat and simmer until squash is tender, about 20 minutes.
3. Puree the soup with an immersion blender or in batches in a regular blender until smooth.
4. Season with salt and pepper, and serve hot.

Nutrition Info Per Serving:

- Calories: 160
- Fat: 5g
- Carbohydrates: 28g
- Protein: 3g
- Fiber: 5g

Serves: 4 **Cooking Time:** 30 minutes

8. Chicken Zoodle Soup
Ingredients:

- 2 tablespoons olive oil
- 1 onion, chopped
- 2 carrots, peeled and diced
- 2 celery stalks, diced
- 2 garlic cloves, minced
- 6 cups chicken broth
- 2 cups cooked chicken, shredded
- 2 zucchinis, spiralized into noodles
- Salt and pepper, to taste

Instructions:

1. In a large pot, heat olive oil over medium heat. Add onion, carrots, celery, and garlic. Cook until vegetables are tender, about 5 minutes.
2. Add chicken broth and bring to a boil. Reduce heat and simmer for 15 minutes.
3. Add cooked chicken and zucchini noodles. Cook for an additional 5 minutes.
4. Season with salt and pepper, and serve hot.

Nutrition Info Per Serving:

- Calories: 210
- Fat: 8g
- Carbohydrates: 15g
- Protein: 20g
- Fiber: 3g

Serves: 4 **Cooking Time:** 25 minutes

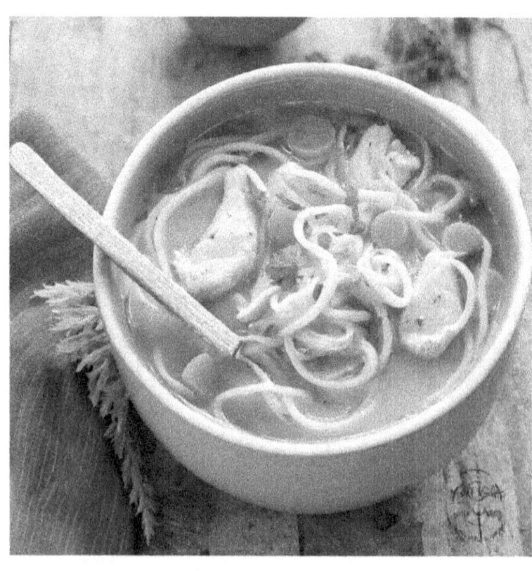

9. Creamy Avocado Cucumber Soup

Ingredients:

- 2 ripe avocados, peeled and pitted
- 1 cucumber, peeled and chopped
- 2 cups plain yogurt
- Juice of 1 lime
- 1 clove garlic, minced
- 1/4 cup fresh cilantro, chopped
- Salt and pepper, to taste
- 1 cup water or vegetable broth, as needed for thinning

Instructions:

1. Combine avocados, cucumber, yogurt, lime juice, garlic, and cilantro in a blender.
2. Blend until smooth, adding water or broth as necessary to reach desired consistency.
3. Season with salt and pepper.
4. Chill for at least 15 minutes before serving.

Nutrition Info Per Serving:

- Calories: 230
- Fat: 15g
- Carbohydrates: 18g
- Protein: 10g
- Fiber: 7g

Serves: 4 **Cooking Time:** 15 minutes (plus chilling)

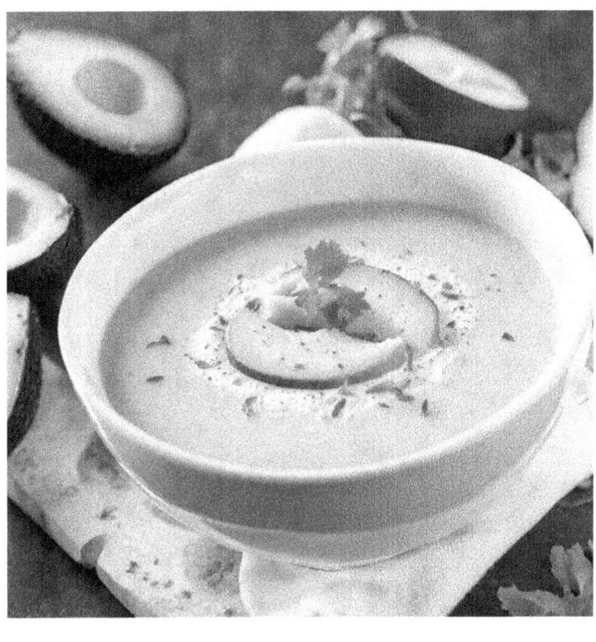

10. Beet and Ginger Soup

Ingredients:

- 3 medium beets, peeled and diced
- 1 tablespoon olive oil
- 1 onion, chopped
- 2 tablespoons grated fresh ginger
- 4 cups vegetable broth
- Salt and pepper, to taste

Instructions:

1. In a pot, heat olive oil over medium heat. Add onion and ginger and cook until onion is translucent, about 5 minutes.
2. Add diced beets and vegetable broth. Bring to a boil, then reduce heat and simmer until beets are tender, about 20 minutes.
3. Puree the soup using an immersion blender or in batches with a regular blender until smooth.
4. Season with salt and pepper, and serve hot.

Nutrition Info Per Serving:

- Calories: 120
- Fat: 3g
- Carbohydrates: 20g
- Protein: 3g
- Fiber: 4g

Serves: 4 Cooking Time: 30 minutes

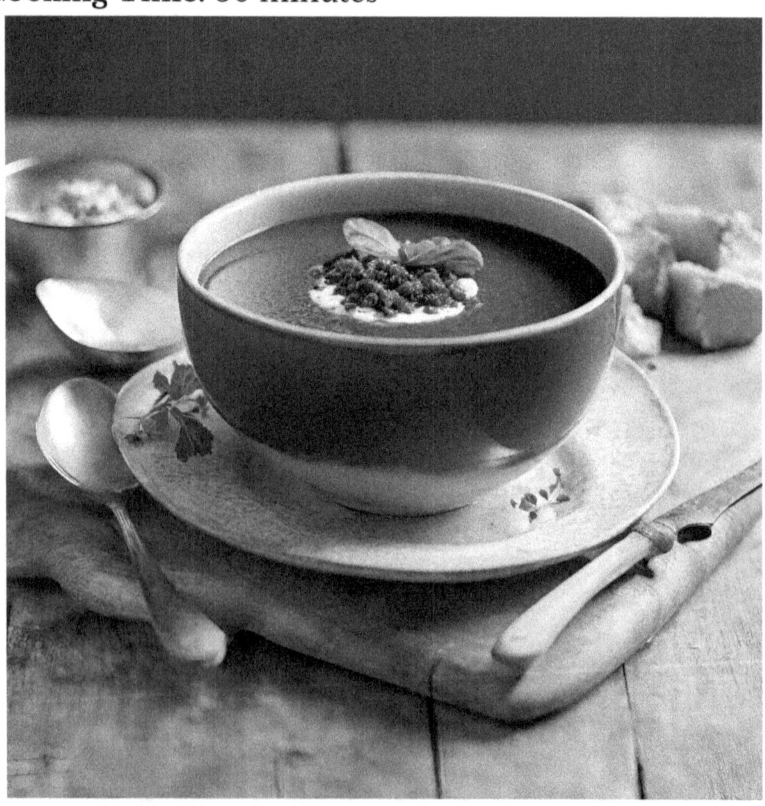

11. Miso Soup with Mushrooms

Ingredients:

- 4 cups water
- 1/4 cup miso paste
- 1 onion, sliced
- 2 cups sliced mushrooms (shiitake or your choice)
- 1/2 cup tofu, cubed
- 2 tablespoons green onions, chopped
- Seaweed (optional), for garnish

Instructions:

1. Bring water to a boil in a pot. Reduce heat to low.
2. Add sliced onion and mushrooms, simmer for about 10 minutes.
3. Dissolve miso paste in a small amount of the hot broth, then stir the mixture back into the pot. Avoid boiling after adding miso to preserve its flavor and nutritional benefits.
4. Add tofu and simmer for another 5 minutes.
5. Garnish with green onions and seaweed if using. Serve hot.

Nutrition Info Per Serving:

- Calories: 80
- Fat: 3g
- Carbohydrates: 10g
- Protein: 6g
- Fiber: 2g

Serves: 4 **Cooking Time:** 20 minutes

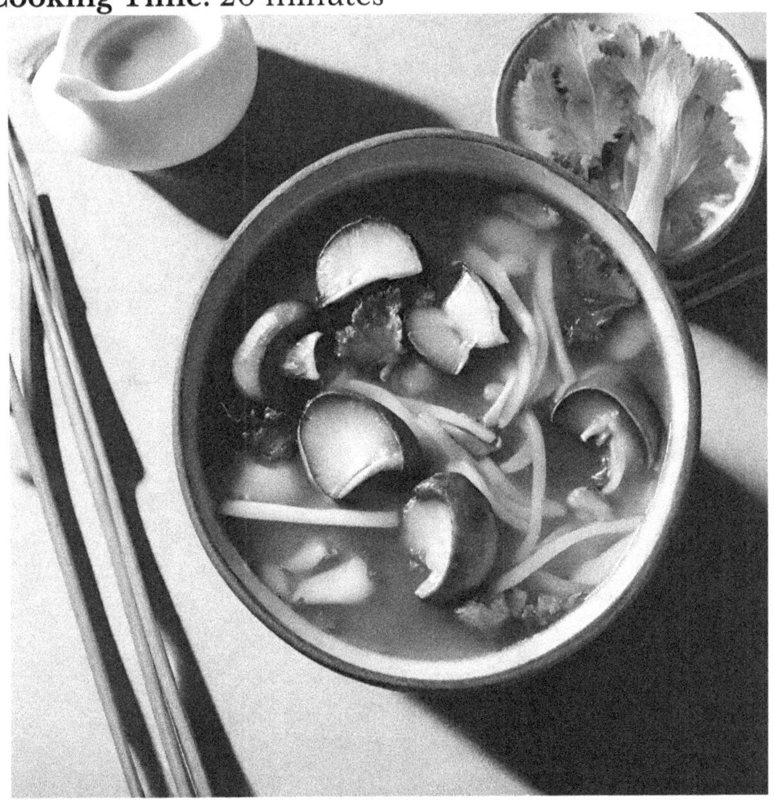

12. Sardine and Arugula Salad

Ingredients:

- 2 cans sardines in olive oil, drained
- 4 cups arugula
- 1/4 cup sliced red onions
- 1/4 cup capers
- Juice of 1 lemon
- 2 tablespoons olive oil
- Salt and pepper, to taste

Instructions:

1. In a salad bowl, combine arugula, red onions, and capers.
2. Top with sardines.
3. In a small bowl, whisk together lemon juice and olive oil, season with salt and pepper.
4. Drizzle the dressing over the salad and toss gently.
5. Serve immediately.

Nutrition Info Per Serving:

- Calories: 220
- Fat: 14g
- Carbohydrates: 4g
- Protein: 20g
- Fiber: 2g

Serves: 4 **Cooking Time:** 10 minutes

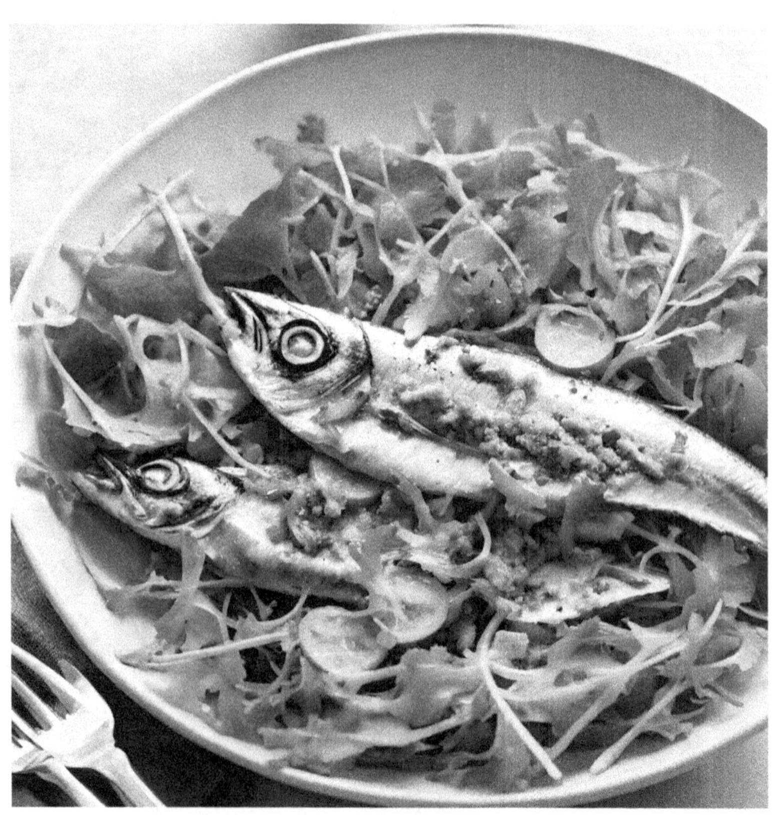

13. Beetroot and Goat Cheese Salad

Ingredients:
- 3 medium beets, roasted, peeled, and sliced
- 1/4 cup crumbled goat cheese
- 1/4 cup walnuts, toasted
- 4 cups mixed greens (such as spinach and arugula)
- For the dressing:
  - 3 tablespoons olive oil
  - 1 tablespoon balsamic vinegar
  - 1 teaspoon honey
  - Salt and pepper, to taste

Instructions:
1. Arrange mixed greens on a platter.
2. Top with sliced beets, crumbled goat cheese, and toasted walnuts.
3. In a small bowl, whisk together olive oil, balsamic vinegar, honey, salt, and pepper to create the dressing.
4. Drizzle the dressing over the salad before serving.

Nutrition Info Per Serving:
- Calories: 250
- Fat: 20g
- Carbohydrates: 15g
- Protein: 7g
- Fiber: 3g

Serves: 4 **Cooking Time:** 15 minutes (excluding beet roasting time)

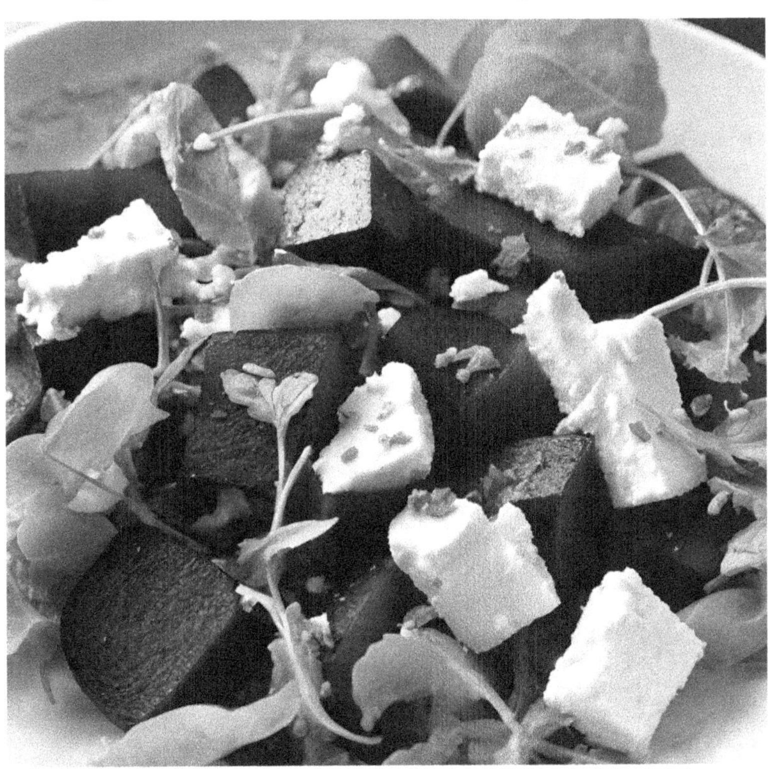

14. Sweet Potato and Lentil Soup

Ingredients:

- 2 tablespoons olive oil
- 1 onion, diced
- 2 cloves garlic, minced
- 1 teaspoon ground cumin
- 1 teaspoon curry powder
- 2 medium sweet potatoes, peeled and diced
- 1 cup red lentils
- 6 cups vegetable broth
- Salt and pepper, to taste
- Fresh cilantro, for garnish

Instructions:

1. Heat olive oil in a large pot over medium heat. Add onion and garlic; cook until softened.
2. Stir in cumin and curry powder; cook for 1 minute.
3. Add sweet potatoes, red lentils, and vegetable broth. Bring to a boil, then simmer for 20 minutes, or until lentils and potatoes are tender.
4. Puree the soup until smooth using an immersion blender or in batches with a regular blender.
5. Season with salt and pepper. Serve garnished with cilantro.

Nutrition Info Per Serving:

- Calories: 210
- Fat: 5g
- Carbohydrates: 35g
- Protein: 8g
- Fiber: 8g

Serves: 4 Cooking Time: 30 minutes

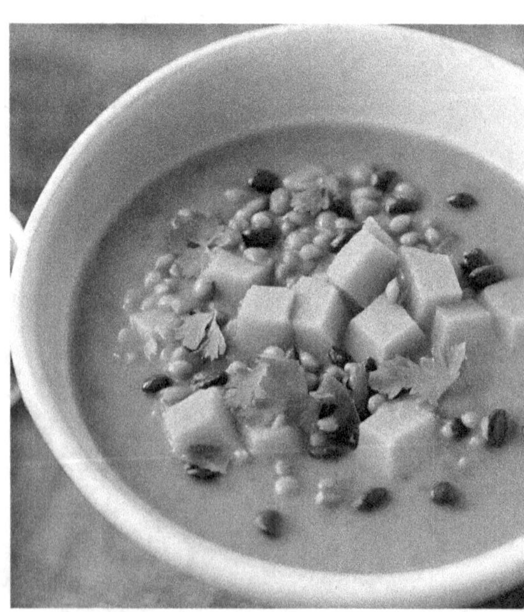

15. Lemon Chicken Orzo Soup

Ingredients:

- 2 tablespoons olive oil
- 1 onion, chopped
- 2 carrots, diced
- 2 stalks celery, diced
- 3 cloves garlic, minced
- 6 cups chicken broth
- 2 chicken breasts, cooked and shredded
- 1 cup orzo pasta
- Juice and zest of 1 lemon
- 2 tablespoons fresh parsley, chopped
- Salt and pepper, to taste

Instructions:

1. In a large pot, heat olive oil over medium heat. Add onion, carrots, celery, and garlic; sauté until vegetables are tender.
2. Add chicken broth and bring to a boil. Add orzo and cook for 10 minutes.
3. Stir in shredded chicken, lemon juice, and zest; cook until heated through.
4. Season with salt and pepper. Stir in parsley just before serving.

Nutrition Info Per Serving:

- Calories: 295
- Fat: 8g
- Carbohydrates: 33g
- Protein: 25g
- Fiber: 3g

Serves: 4 **Cooking Time:** 30 minutes

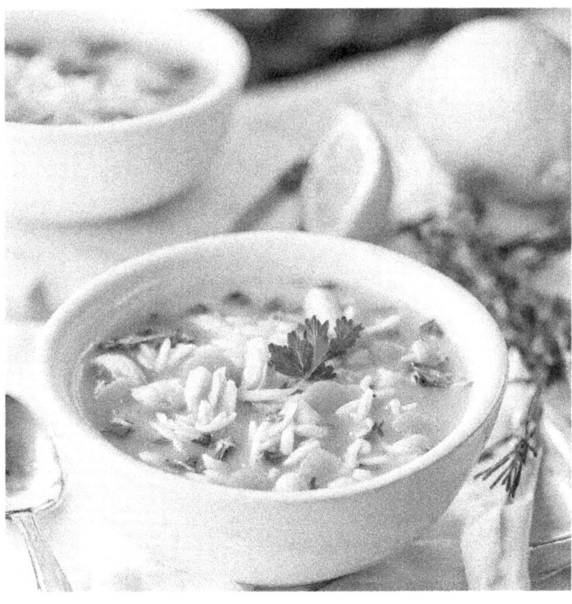

16. Coconut Shrimp Soup

Ingredients:

- 1 tablespoon coconut oil
- 1 onion, chopped
- 2 cloves garlic, minced
- 1 red bell pepper, diced
- 1 tablespoon grated ginger
- 1 can (14 oz) coconut milk
- 4 cups vegetable broth
- 1 pound shrimp, peeled and deveined
- Juice of 1 lime
- 1/4 cup chopped fresh cilantro
- Salt and pepper, to taste

Instructions:

1. In a large pot, heat coconut oil over medium heat. Add onion, garlic, bell pepper, and ginger; cook until vegetables are soft.
2. Pour in coconut milk and vegetable broth, and bring to a simmer.
3. Add shrimp and cook until they are pink and cooked through, about 5 minutes.
4. Stir in lime juice and cilantro. Season with salt and pepper.
5. Serve hot.

Nutrition Info Per Serving:

- Calories: 300
- Fat: 18g
- Carbohydrates: 15g
- Protein: 20g
- Fiber: 2g

Serves: 4 **Cooking Time:** 25 minutes

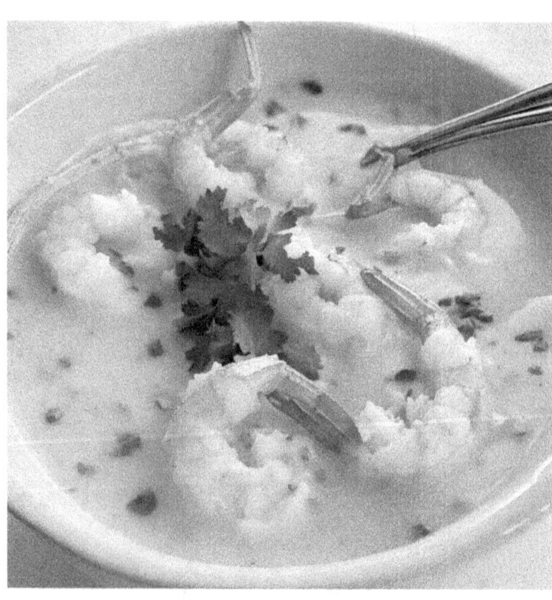

17. Broccoli Almond Soup

Ingredients:

- 1 tablespoon olive oil
- 1 onion, chopped
- 2 cloves garlic, minced
- 4 cups broccoli florets
- 4 cups vegetable broth
- 1/2 cup ground almonds
- Salt and pepper, to taste

Instructions:

1. In a large pot, heat olive oil over medium heat. Add onion and garlic; sauté until translucent.
2. Add broccoli and broth; bring to a boil. Reduce heat and simmer until broccoli is tender, about 15 minutes.
3. Stir in ground almonds, and continue to cook for 5 minutes.
4. Puree the soup until smooth using an immersion blender or in batches with a regular blender.
5. Season with salt and pepper. Serve hot.

Nutrition Info Per Serving:

- Calories: 190
- Fat: 12g
- Carbohydrates: 15g
- Protein: 7g
- Fiber: 5g

Serves: 4 **Cooking Time:** 25 minutes

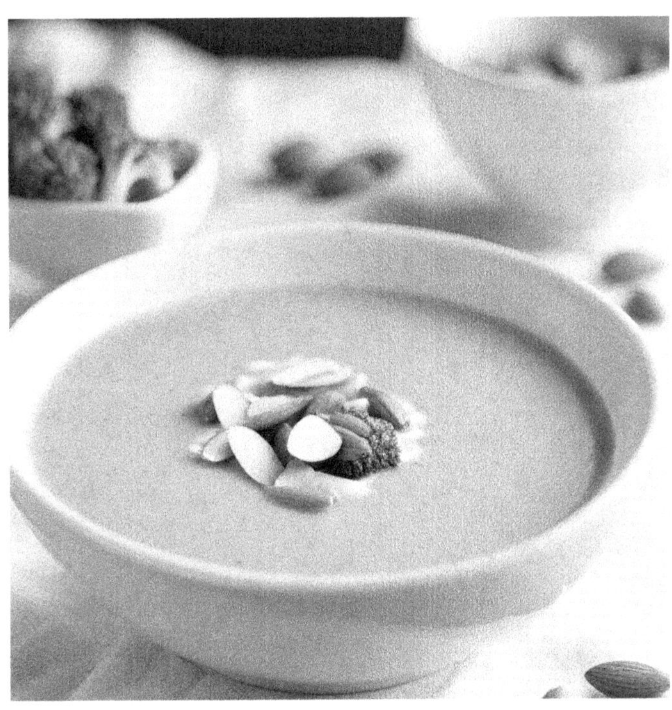

18. Turkey Cobb Salad

Ingredients:

- 4 cups chopped Romaine lettuce
- 2 cups cooked turkey breast, diced
- 4 hard-boiled eggs, peeled and quartered
- 1 avocado, diced
- 1 cup cherry tomatoes, halved
- 1/2 cup crumbled blue cheese
- 1/2 cup cooked bacon, crumbled
- For the dressing:
    - 1/4 cup olive oil
    - 2 tablespoons red wine vinegar
    - 1 teaspoon Dijon mustard
    - Salt and pepper, to taste

Instructions:

1. Arrange Romaine lettuce on a large platter.
2. Neatly arrange rows of turkey, eggs, avocado, tomatoes, blue cheese, and bacon over the lettuce.
3. In a small bowl, whisk together olive oil, red wine vinegar, Dijon mustard, salt, and pepper to make the dressing.
4. Drizzle the dressing over the salad just before serving.

Nutrition Info Per Serving:

- Calories: 450
- Fat: 30g
- Carbohydrates: 12g
- Protein: 35g
- Fiber: 5g

Serves: 4 Cooking Time: 15 minutes (excluding cooking time for turkey and eggs if not pre-prepared)

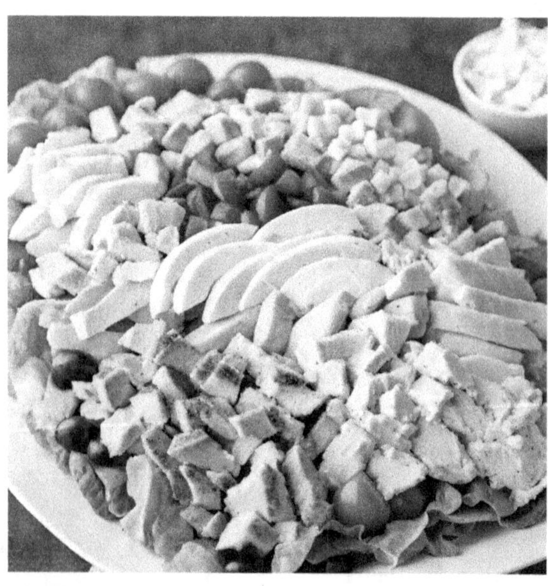

19. Asian Chicken Salad

Ingredients:

- 4 cups mixed greens
- 2 cups cooked chicken breast, shredded
- 1 cup shredded carrots
- 1 red bell pepper, sliced thin
- 1/2 cup sliced almonds, toasted
- 1/4 cup cilantro, chopped
- For the dressing:
    - 3 tablespoons soy sauce
    - 2 tablespoons sesame oil
    - 1 tablespoon honey
    - 1 garlic clove, minced
    - 1 teaspoon grated ginger

Instructions:

1. In a large salad bowl, combine mixed greens, chicken, carrots, red bell pepper, almonds, and cilantro.
2. In a small bowl, whisk together soy sauce, sesame oil, honey, minced garlic, and ginger to make the dressing.
3. Pour the dressing over the salad and toss to coat evenly.
4. Serve immediately.

Nutrition Info Per Serving:

- Calories: 320
- Fat: 18g
- Carbohydrates: 12g
- Protein: 28g
- Fiber: 4g

Serves: 4 **Cooking Time:** 10 minutes

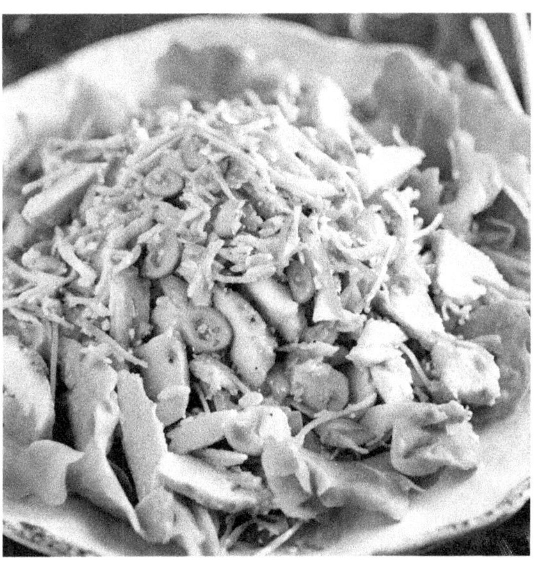

20. Tuna Salad Nicoise

Ingredients:

- 4 cups mixed salad greens
- 2 cans (6 oz each) tuna in olive oil, drained and flaked
- 4 small new potatoes, boiled and quartered
- 2 hard-boiled eggs, peeled and quartered
- 1/2 cup green beans, trimmed and blanched
- 1/4 cup black olives, pitted
- For the dressing:
  - 1/4 cup olive oil
  - 2 tablespoons lemon juice
  - 1 tablespoon Dijon mustard
  - Salt and pepper, to taste

Instructions:

1. Arrange salad greens on a large platter.
2. Top with separate piles of tuna, potatoes, eggs, green beans, and olives.
3. In a small bowl, whisk together olive oil, lemon juice, Dijon mustard, salt, and pepper to make the dressing.
4. Drizzle the dressing over the salad before serving.

Nutrition Info Per Serving:

- Calories: 360
- Fat: 20g
- Carbohydrates: 20g
- Protein: 25g
- Fiber: 4g

Serves: 4 **Cooking Time:** 20 minutes (including time for boiling eggs and potatoes)

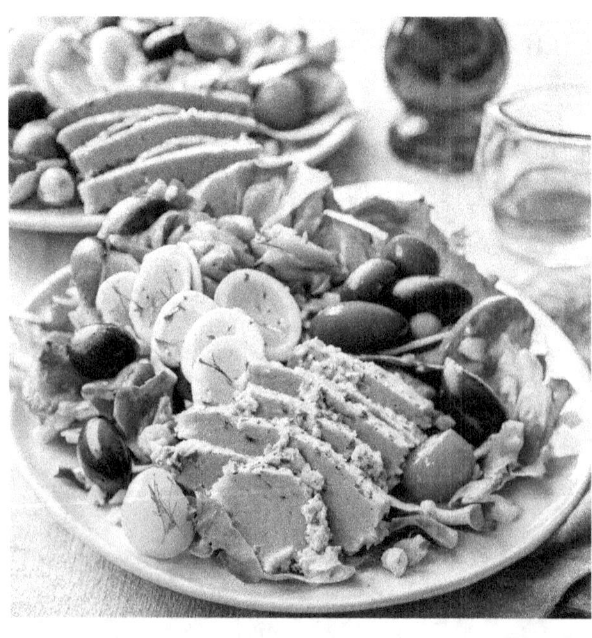

21. Greek Salad with Grilled Chicken

Ingredients:

- 4 cups chopped Romaine lettuce
- 2 cups grilled chicken breast, sliced
- 1 cucumber, sliced
- 1 cup cherry tomatoes, halved
- 1/2 red onion, thinly sliced
- 1/2 cup feta cheese, crumbled
- 1/4 cup Kalamata olives, pitted
- For the dressing:
    - 1/4 cup olive oil
    - 2 tablespoons red wine vinegar
    - 1 teaspoon dried oregano
    - Salt and pepper, to taste

Instructions:

1. In a large salad bowl, combine Romaine lettuce, grilled chicken, cucumber, cherry tomatoes, red onion, feta cheese, and olives.
2. In a small bowl, whisk together olive oil, red wine vinegar, oregano, salt, and pepper to make the dressing.
3. Pour the dressing over the salad and toss to combine.
4. Serve chilled.

Nutrition Info Per Serving:

- Calories: 350
- Fat: 20g
- Carbohydrates: 10g
- Protein: 30g
- Fiber: 3g

Serves: 4 **Cooking Time:** 15 minutes

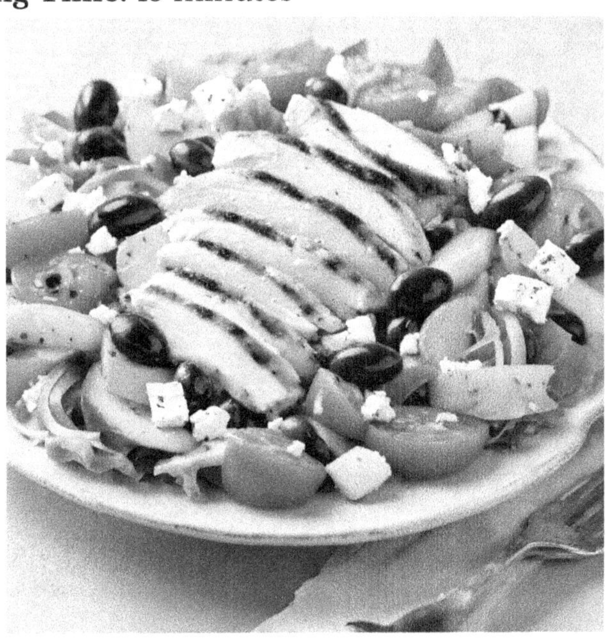

22. Pear and Blue Cheese Salad

Ingredients:

- 4 cups mixed greens
- 2 pears, cored and sliced
- 1/2 cup crumbled blue cheese
- 1/4 cup walnuts, toasted and chopped
- For the dressing:
    - 1/4 cup olive oil
    - 2 tablespoons balsamic vinegar
    - 1 teaspoon honey
    - Salt and pepper, to taste

Instructions:

1. In a salad bowl, arrange mixed greens, pear slices, blue cheese, and walnuts.
2. In a small bowl, whisk together olive oil, balsamic vinegar, honey, salt, and pepper to make the dressing.
3. Drizzle the dressing over the salad and toss gently to combine.
4. Serve immediately.

Nutrition Info Per Serving:

- Calories: 270
- Fat: 20g
- Carbohydrates: 18g
- Protein: 6g
- Fiber: 4g

Serves: 4 Cooking Time: 10 minutes

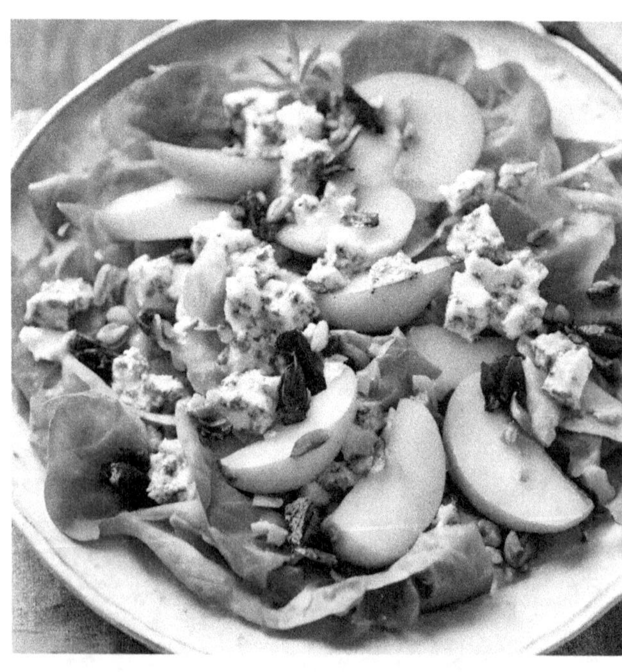

23. Broccoli and Bacon Salad

Ingredients:

- 4 cups fresh broccoli florets
- 6 slices bacon, cooked and crumbled
- 1/4 cup red onion, chopped
- 1/2 cup raisins
- 1/4 cup sunflower seeds
- 3/4 cup mayonnaise
- 2 tablespoons apple cider vinegar
- 1 tablespoon sugar
- Salt and pepper, to taste

Instructions:

1. In a large bowl, combine broccoli, bacon, red onion, raisins, and sunflower seeds.
2. In a small bowl, whisk together mayonnaise, apple cider vinegar, sugar, salt, and pepper to create the dressing.
3. Pour dressing over the broccoli mixture and toss to coat evenly.
4. Chill in the refrigerator for at least 15 minutes before serving.

Nutrition Info Per Serving:

- Calories: 320
- Fat: 24g
- Carbohydrates: 22g
- Protein: 8g
- Fiber: 3g

Serves: 4 **Cooking Time:** 15 minutes

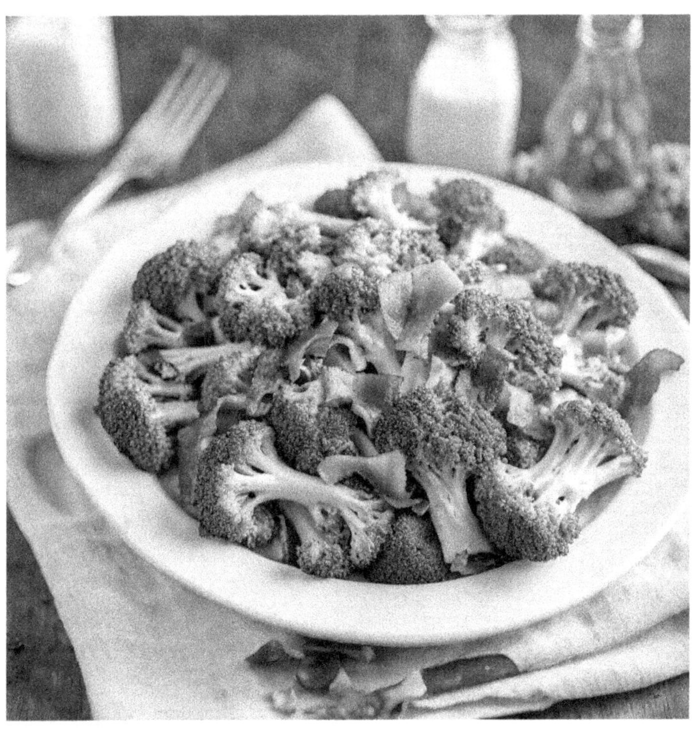

24. Shrimp and Avocado Salad

Ingredients:

- 1 pound cooked shrimp, peeled and deveined
- 2 avocados, diced
- 1/4 cup red onion, finely chopped
- 1/4 cup cilantro, chopped
- Juice of 2 limes
- 2 tablespoons olive oil
- Salt and pepper, to taste

Instructions:

1. In a large bowl, combine shrimp, avocados, red onion, and cilantro.
2. In a small bowl, whisk together lime juice, olive oil, salt, and pepper to create the dressing.
3. Drizzle dressing over the salad and gently toss to combine.
4. Serve immediately or chill until ready to serve.

Nutrition Info Per Serving:

- Calories: 290
- Fat: 20g
- Carbohydrates: 10g
- Protein: 20g
- Fiber: 7g

Serves: 4 **Cooking Time:** 10 minutes

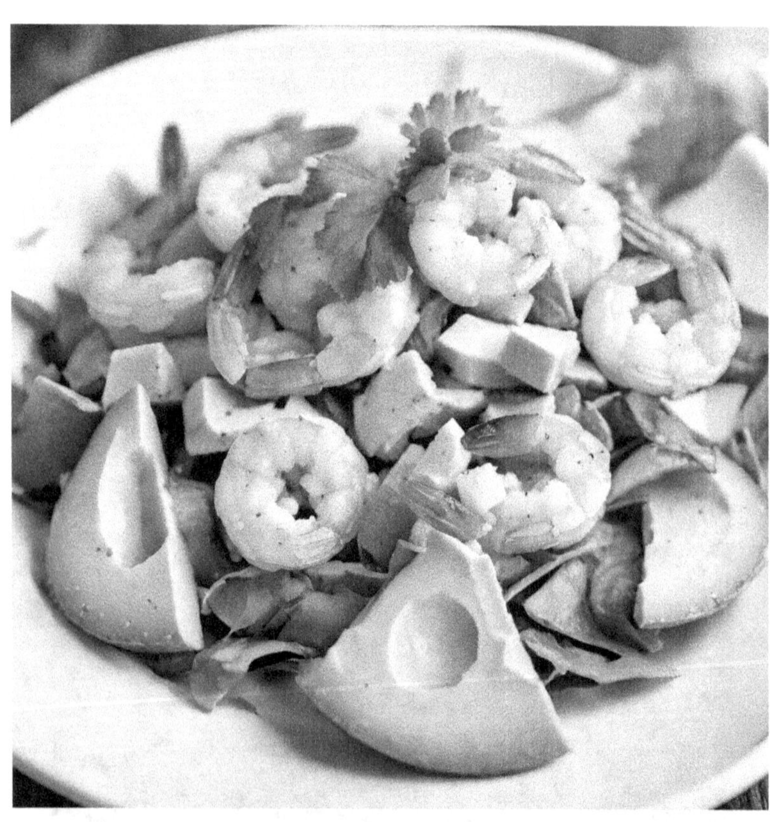

25. Endive and Apple Salad

Ingredients:

- 3 endives, trimmed and leaves separated
- 2 apples, cored and thinly sliced
- 1/4 cup walnuts, chopped
- 1/4 cup blue cheese, crumbled
- 3 tablespoons olive oil
- 1 tablespoon apple cider vinegar
- 1 teaspoon honey
- Salt and pepper, to taste

Instructions:

1. Arrange endive leaves and apple slices in a salad bowl.
2. Sprinkle with walnuts and blue cheese.
3. In a small bowl, whisk together olive oil, apple cider vinegar, honey, salt, and pepper to make the dressing.
4. Drizzle the dressing over the salad and toss lightly.
5. Serve immediately.

Nutrition Info Per Serving:

- Calories: 220
- Fat: 17g
- Carbohydrates: 14g
- Protein: 4g
- Fiber: 3g

Serves: 4 **Cooking Time:** 10 minutes

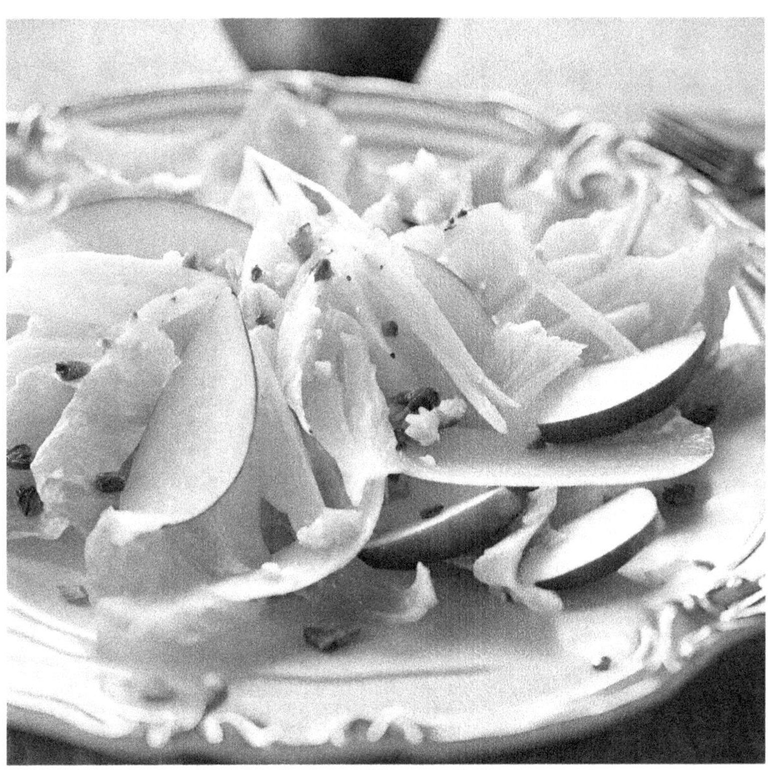

26. Carrot and Raisin Salad

Ingredients:

- 4 cups shredded carrots
- 1/2 cup raisins
- 1/4 cup plain yogurt
- 2 tablespoons honey
- 1 tablespoon lemon juice
- Salt and pepper, to taste

Instructions:

1. In a large bowl, combine shredded carrots and raisins.
2. In a small bowl, mix yogurt, honey, lemon juice, salt, and pepper to create the dressing.
3. Pour dressing over the carrot mixture and toss to combine.
4. Chill in the refrigerator for at least 10 minutes before serving.

Nutrition Info Per Serving:

- Calories: 150
- Fat: 1g
- Carbohydrates: 35g
- Protein: 2g
- Fiber: 4g

Serves: 4 Cooking Time: 10 minutes

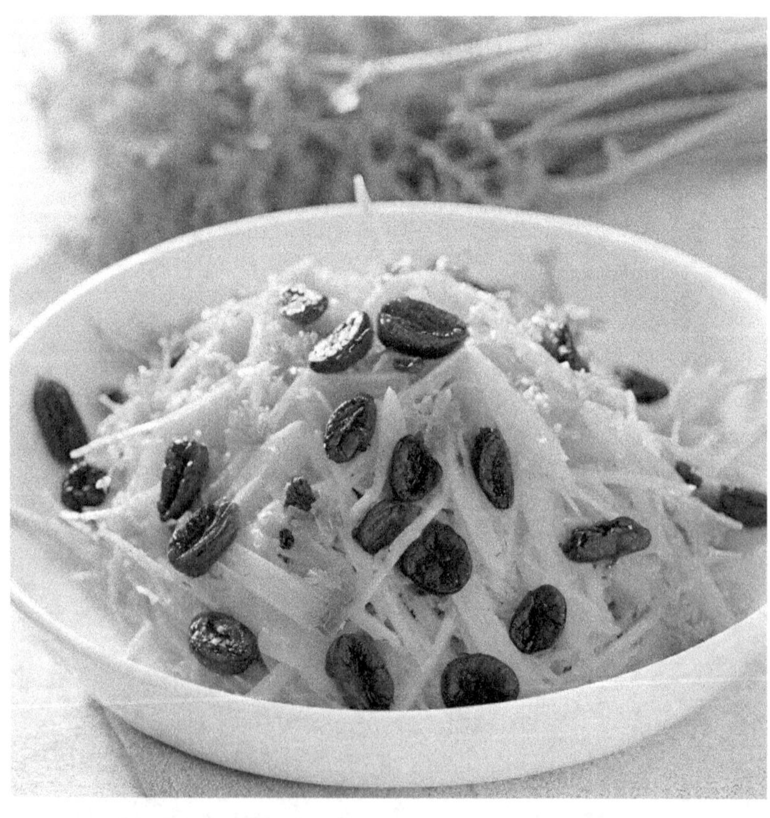

27. Radish and Spring Onion Salad

Ingredients:

- 2 cups sliced radishes
- 1 cup chopped spring onions
- 1/4 cup chopped fresh parsley
- 2 tablespoons olive oil
- 1 tablespoon white wine vinegar
- Salt and pepper, to taste

Instructions:

1. In a salad bowl, combine radishes, spring onions, and parsley.
2. In a small bowl, whisk together olive oil, vinegar, salt, and pepper to make the dressing.
3. Drizzle the dressing over the salad and toss well.
4. Serve chilled or at room temperature.

Nutrition Info Per Serving:

- Calories: 100
- Fat: 7g
- Carbohydrates: 8g
- Protein: 1g
- Fiber: 2g

Serves: 4 **Cooking Time:** 10 minutes

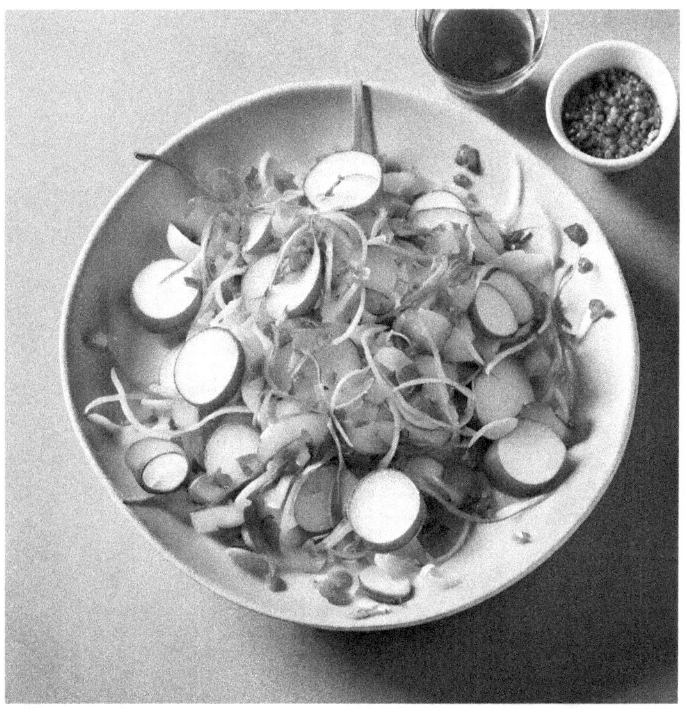

Poultry & Meat Recipes

1. Lemon Herb Chicken Breast

Ingredients:

- 4 boneless, skinless chicken breasts
- 2 lemons, zest and juice
- 2 tablespoons olive oil
- 2 cloves garlic, minced
- 1 teaspoon dried thyme
- 1 teaspoon dried rosemary
- Salt and pepper, to taste

Instructions:

1. In a small bowl, mix lemon zest, lemon juice, olive oil, garlic, thyme, rosemary, salt, and pepper.
2. Place chicken breasts in a shallow dish and pour the marinade over them. Let marinate for at least 15 minutes in the refrigerator.
3. Preheat a grill or skillet over medium heat.
4. Remove chicken from marinade and cook for 6-7 minutes per side or until fully cooked and juices run clear.
5. Serve garnished with lemon slices.

Nutrition Info Per Serving:

- Calories: 230
- Fat: 10g
- Carbohydrates: 3g
- Protein: 30g
- Fiber: 0g

Serves: 4 Cooking Time: 20 minutes

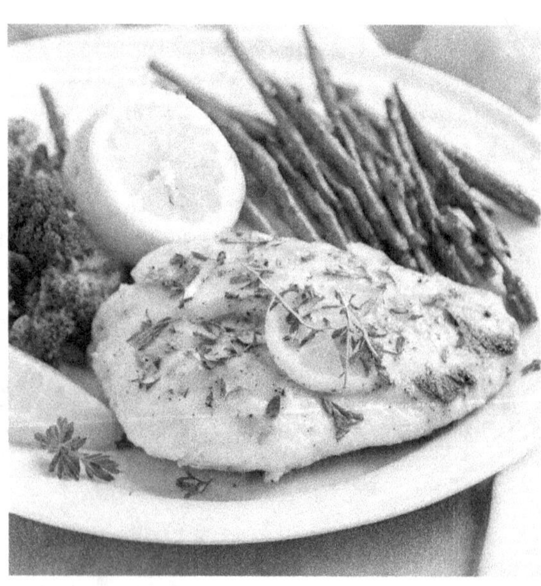

2. Turkey Patties with Sage

Ingredients:

- 1 pound ground turkey
- 1/4 cup finely chopped onion
- 2 cloves garlic, minced
- 2 tablespoons chopped fresh sage
- 1 egg, beaten
- Salt and pepper, to taste
- 1 tablespoon olive oil

Instructions:

1. In a large bowl, combine ground turkey, onion, garlic, sage, egg, salt, and pepper.
2. Form the mixture into 4 patties.
3. Heat olive oil in a skillet over medium heat.
4. Cook patties for about 5-6 minutes per side or until cooked through and golden brown.
5. Serve hot.

Nutrition Info Per Serving:

- Calories: 220
- Fat: 12g
- Carbohydrates: 2g
- Protein: 26g
- Fiber: 0g

Serves: 4 **Cooking Time:** 20 minutes

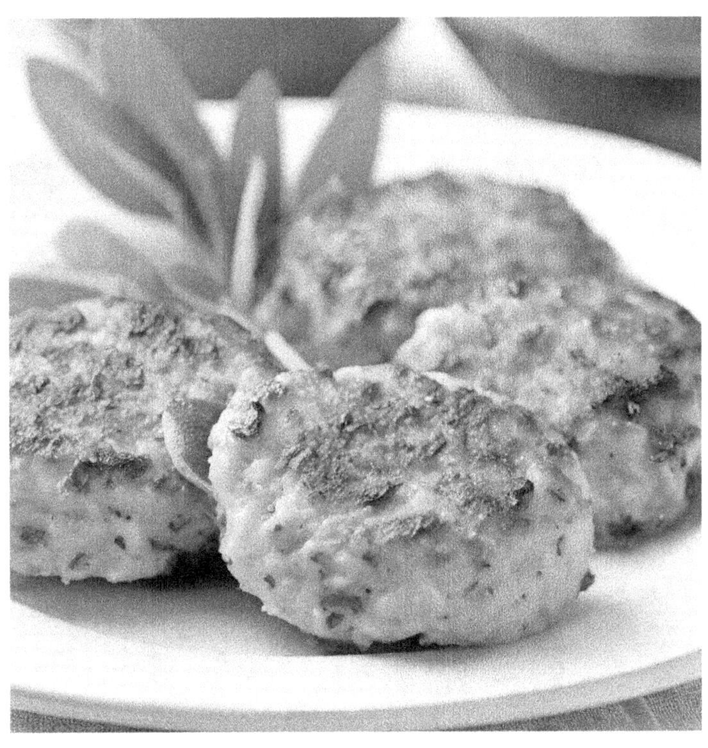

3. Beef and Broccoli Stir-Fry

Ingredients:

- 1 pound flank steak, thinly sliced
- 3 cups broccoli florets
- 2 tablespoons vegetable oil
- 2 cloves garlic, minced
- For the sauce:
  - 1/3 cup soy sauce
  - 1/4 cup water
  - 1 tablespoon cornstarch
  - 1 tablespoon honey
  - 1 teaspoon sesame oil

Instructions:

1. In a small bowl, whisk together soy sauce, water, cornstarch, honey, and sesame oil to make the sauce.
2. Heat 1 tablespoon of vegetable oil in a large skillet or wok over medium-high heat.
3. Add broccoli and stir-fry until tender-crisp, about 3 minutes. Remove from skillet and set aside.
4. Add the remaining oil to the skillet. Add garlic and sliced steak, stir-frying until the steak is nearly cooked through, about 3-4 minutes.
5. Return the broccoli to the skillet and pour the sauce over the top. Cook, stirring, until the sauce has thickened and the steak is fully cooked, about 2 minutes.
6. Serve immediately.

Nutrition Info Per Serving:

- Calories: 280
- Fat: 15g
- Carbohydrates: 12g
- Protein: 26g
- Fiber: 2g

Serves: 4 Cooking Time: 20 minutes

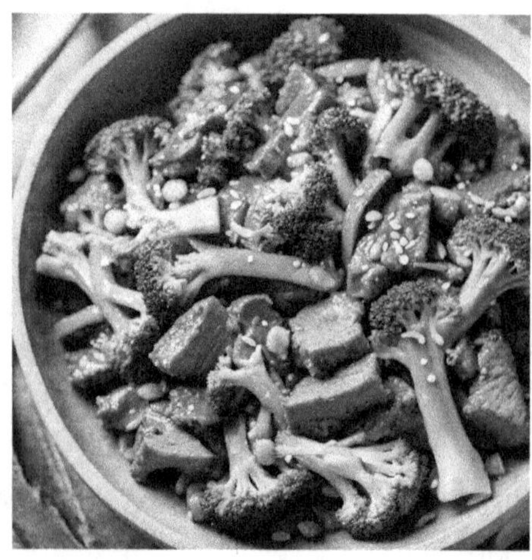

4. Lamb Chops with Rosemary

Ingredients:

- 8 lamb chops
- 2 tablespoons olive oil
- 2 cloves garlic, minced
- 2 tablespoons fresh rosemary, chopped
- Salt and pepper, to taste

Instructions:

1. Rub each lamb chop with olive oil, garlic, rosemary, salt, and pepper.
2. Preheat a grill or skillet over medium-high heat.
3. Cook lamb chops for about 3-4 minutes per side for medium-rare, or longer depending on desired doneness.
4. Let rest for a few minutes before serving.

Nutrition Info Per Serving:

- Calories: 350
- Fat: 25g
- Carbohydrates: 0g
- Protein: 30g
- Fiber: 0g

Serves: 4 (2 chops each) **Cooking Time:** 15 minutes

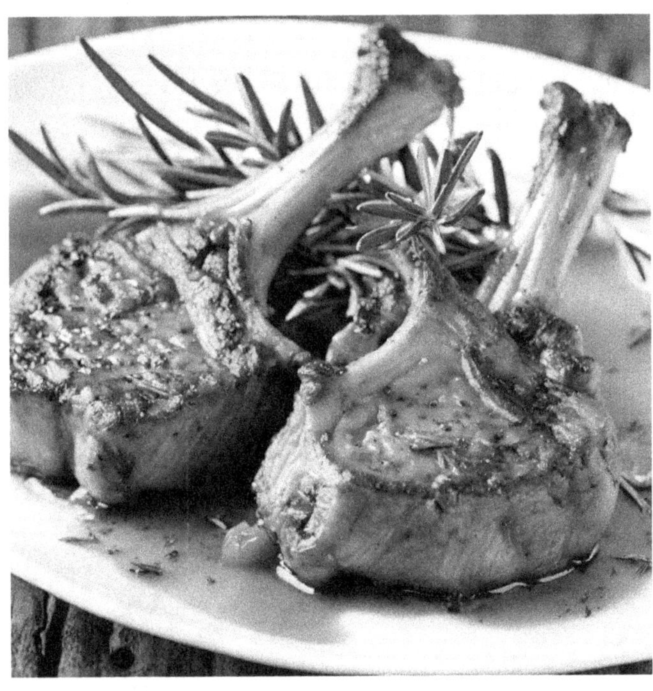

5. Spiced Chicken Stir-Fry

Ingredients:

- 1 pound chicken breast, thinly sliced
- 2 tablespoons vegetable oil
- 1 bell pepper, sliced
- 1 onion, sliced
- 2 cloves garlic, minced
- 1 tablespoon ginger, minced
- 2 teaspoons cumin
- 2 teaspoons paprika
- 1 teaspoon turmeric
- Salt and pepper, to taste
- 2 tablespoons soy sauce
- 1 tablespoon honey

Instructions:

1. Heat oil in a large skillet over medium-high heat. Add chicken and stir-fry until it starts to brown, about 5 minutes.
2. Add bell pepper, onion, garlic, and ginger, and cook for another 5 minutes.
3. Sprinkle cumin, paprika, and turmeric over the chicken and vegetables. Stir to coat evenly.
4. Drizzle soy sauce and honey over the chicken and vegetables. Stir well and cook for another 5 minutes, until everything is cooked through and well coated.
5. Season with salt and pepper to taste. Serve hot.

Nutrition Info Per Serving:

- Calories: 265
- Fat: 9g
- Carbohydrates: 15g
- Protein: 30g
- Fiber: 2g

Serves: 4 **Cooking Time:** 20 minutes

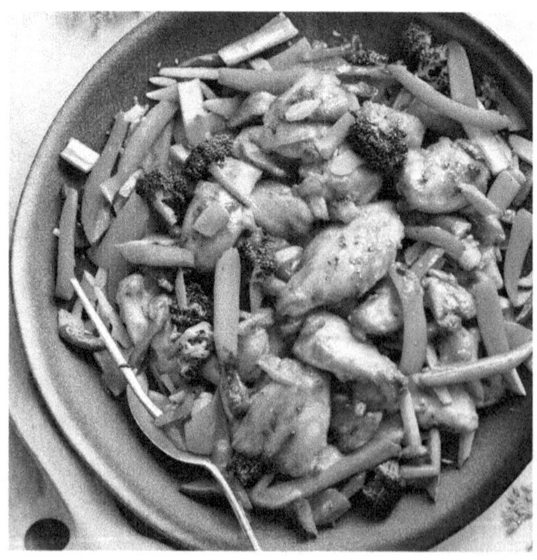

6. Basil Pesto Chicken

Ingredients:

- 4 boneless, skinless chicken breasts
- Salt and pepper, to taste
- 1/2 cup basil pesto
- 2 tablespoons olive oil

Instructions:

1. Season chicken breasts with salt and pepper.
2. Spread basil pesto evenly over each chicken breast.
3. Heat olive oil in a skillet over medium heat. Add chicken and cook for 6-7 minutes on each side, until cooked through and golden on the outside.
4. Serve hot, topped with additional pesto if desired.

Nutrition Info Per Serving:

- Calories: 330
- Fat: 20g
- Carbohydrates: 3g
- Protein: 34g
- Fiber: 1g

Serves: 4 **Cooking Time:** 15 minutes

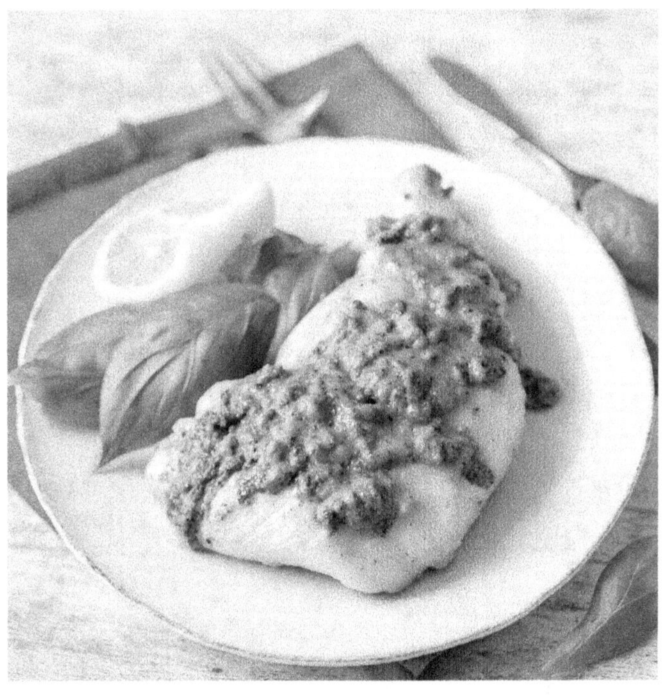

7. Chicken Caesar Salad

Ingredients:

- 2 romaine lettuce heads, chopped
- 1 pound grilled chicken breast, sliced
- 1 cup croutons
- 1/2 cup grated Parmesan cheese
- Caesar dressing (commercial or homemade)
- Lemon wedges, for serving

Instructions:

1. In a large salad bowl, combine chopped lettuce, sliced grilled chicken, croutons, and Parmesan cheese.
2. Drizzle Caesar dressing over the salad and toss to combine.
3. Serve with lemon wedges on the side.

Nutrition Info Per Serving:

- Calories: 320
- Fat: 16g
- Carbohydrates: 12g
- Protein: 32g
- Fiber: 3g

Serves: 4 **Cooking Time:** 10 minutes (if chicken is pre-cooked)

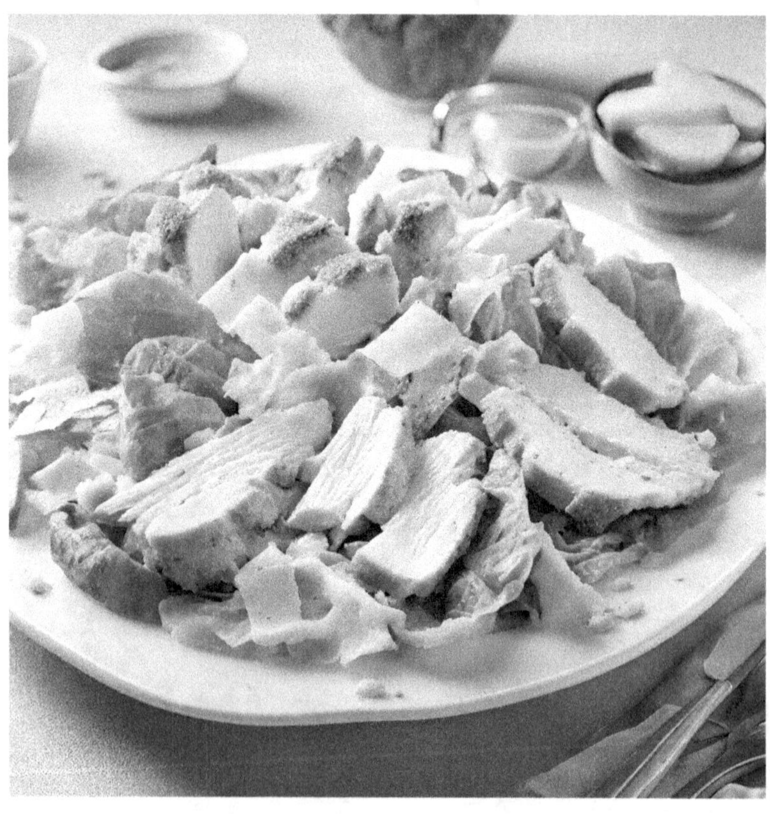

8. Buffalo Chicken Lettuce Wraps

Ingredients:

- 1 pound cooked chicken breast, shredded
- 1/2 cup buffalo sauce
- 1 head iceberg lettuce, leaves separated
- 1/2 cup blue cheese, crumbled
- 1/4 cup chopped celery
- 1/4 cup chopped carrots

Instructions:

1. In a bowl, mix the shredded chicken with buffalo sauce.
2. Place a spoonful of chicken mixture into each lettuce leaf.
3. Top with blue cheese, celery, and carrots.
4. Serve the lettuce wraps immediately.

Nutrition Info Per Serving:

- Calories: 215
- Fat: 8g
- Carbohydrates: 5g
- Protein: 29g
- Fiber: 2g

Serves: 4 **Cooking Time:** 10 minutes

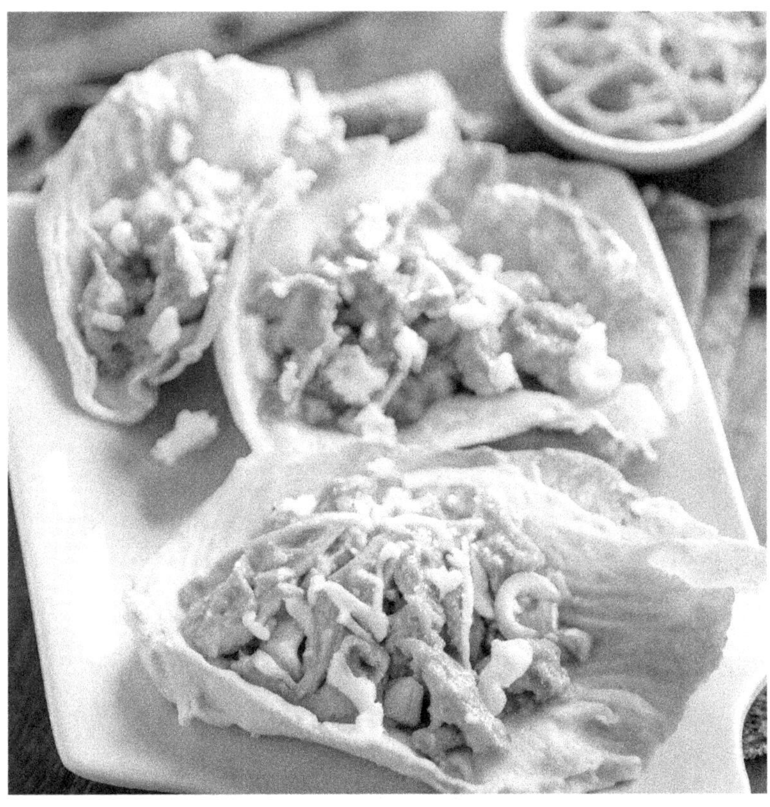

9. Greek Lemon Chicken Skewers

Ingredients:

- 1 pound chicken breast, cut into cubes
- 3 tablespoons olive oil
- Juice and zest of 1 lemon
- 2 cloves garlic, minced
- 1 tablespoon dried oregano
- Salt and pepper, to taste

Instructions:

1. In a bowl, combine olive oil, lemon juice and zest, garlic, oregano, salt, and pepper.
2. Add chicken cubes to the marinade and let sit for at least 15 minutes.
3. Preheat a grill or grill pan over medium-high heat.
4. Thread chicken onto skewers and grill for about 10 minutes, turning occasionally, until cooked through.
5. Serve hot.

Nutrition Info Per Serving:

- Calories: 225
- Fat: 10g
- Carbohydrates: 3g
- Protein: 30g
- Fiber: 0g

Serves: 4 Cooking Time: 20 minutes

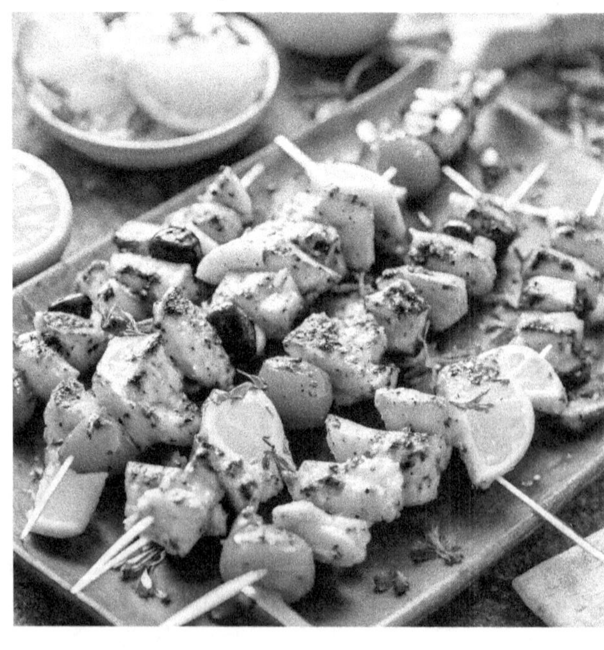

10. Thai Coconut Curry Chicken

Ingredients:

- 1 pound chicken breast, cubed
- 1 tablespoon coconut oil
- 1 onion, chopped
- 2 cloves garlic, minced
- 1 bell pepper, sliced
- 1 tablespoon Thai red curry paste
- 1 can (14 oz) coconut milk
- 1 tablespoon fish sauce
- 1 tablespoon sugar
- Juice of 1 lime
- 1/4 cup fresh basil, chopped
- Salt and pepper, to taste

Instructions:

1. Heat coconut oil in a large skillet over medium heat. Add onion and garlic, and sauté until softened.
2. Add chicken and cook until it is no longer pink.
3. Stir in bell pepper and curry paste, cooking for a few more minutes to release the flavors.
4. Pour in coconut milk, fish sauce, and sugar. Bring to a simmer and cook for about 10 minutes or until the chicken is fully cooked and the sauce has thickened slightly.
5. Finish with lime juice and basil. Season with salt and pepper to taste.
6. Serve hot, ideally over cooked rice or noodles.

Nutrition Info Per Serving:

- Calories: 350
- Fat: 22g
- Carbohydrates: 10g
- Protein: 28g
- Fiber: 1g

Serves: 4 **Cooking Time:** 25 minutes

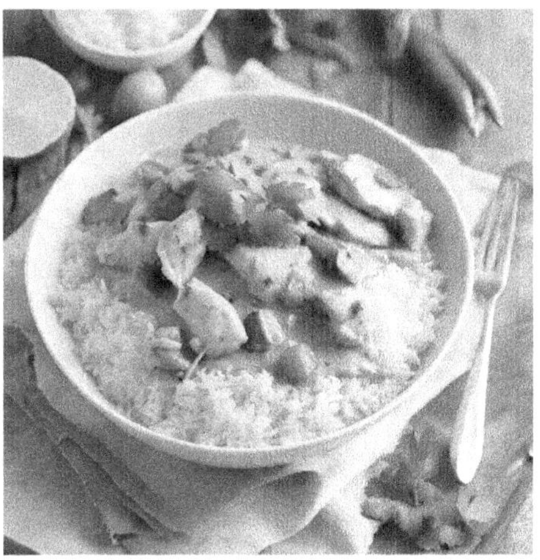

11. Pork Tenderloin with Apples

Ingredients:

- 1 pork tenderloin (about 1 pound)
- Salt and pepper, to taste
- 2 tablespoons olive oil
- 2 apples, sliced
- 1 onion, sliced
- 1/2 cup apple cider
- 1 teaspoon fresh thyme

Instructions:

1. Season the pork tenderloin with salt and pepper.
2. Heat olive oil in a large skillet over medium-high heat. Add the pork and sear on all sides until golden brown.
3. Remove the pork and add apples and onions to the skillet. Cook until they begin to soften.
4. Return the pork to the skillet, add apple cider and thyme. Cover and simmer for about 15 minutes or until the pork reaches an internal temperature of 145°F (63°C).
5. Slice the pork and serve with the apples and onions.

Nutrition Info Per Serving:

- Calories: 280
- Fat: 12g
- Carbohydrates: 15g
- Protein: 28g
- Fiber: 2g

Serves: 4 **Cooking Time:** 30 minutes

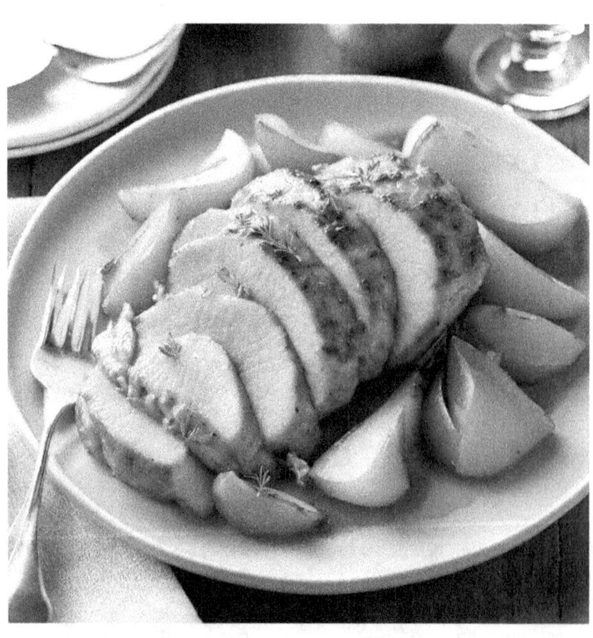

12. Quick Beef Stroganoff

Ingredients:

- 1 pound beef sirloin, thinly sliced
- 2 tablespoons butter
- 1 onion, chopped
- 2 cloves garlic, minced
- 1 cup mushrooms, sliced
- 1 tablespoon all-purpose flour
- 1 cup beef broth
- 1/2 cup sour cream
- Salt and pepper, to taste
- 2 tablespoons fresh parsley, chopped

Instructions:

1. Melt butter in a large skillet over medium-high heat. Add onion, garlic, and mushrooms. Cook until softened.
2. Add beef and cook until browned.
3. Sprinkle flour over the beef and vegetables, stir to coat.
4. Pour in beef broth, bring to a boil, then reduce heat and simmer for about 10 minutes.
5. Stir in sour cream and heat through without boiling. Season with salt and pepper.
6. Garnish with fresh parsley and serve over cooked noodles or rice.

Nutrition Info Per Serving:

- Calories: 320
- Fat: 18g
- Carbohydrates: 8g
- Protein: 30g
- Fiber: 1g

Serves: 4 **Cooking Time:** 25 minutes

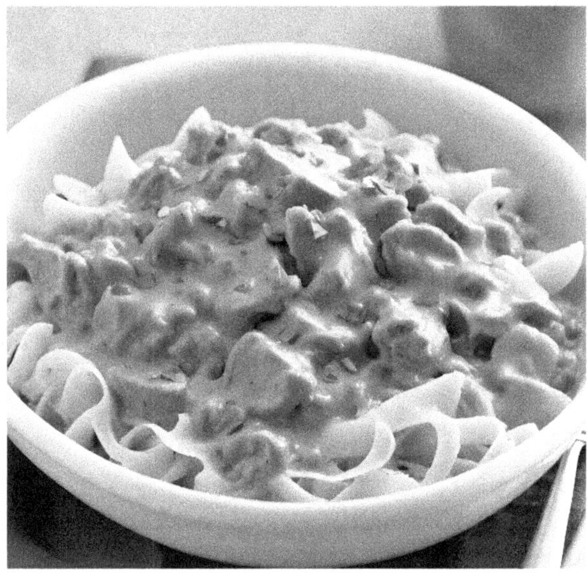

13. Garlic Herb Pork Chops

Ingredients:

- 4 pork chops
- Salt and pepper, to taste
- 2 tablespoons olive oil
- 3 cloves garlic, minced
- 1 teaspoon dried thyme
- 1 teaspoon dried rosemary

Instructions:

1. Season pork chops with salt and pepper.
2. Heat olive oil in a skillet over medium heat. Add pork chops and cook until golden and cooked through, about 5-7 minutes per side.
3. Add garlic, thyme, and rosemary in the last 2 minutes of cooking.
4. Serve the pork chops hot with the garlic and herbs spooned over the top.

Nutrition Info Per Serving:

- Calories: 290
- Fat: 16g
- Carbohydrates: 2g
- Protein: 32g
- Fiber: 0g

Serves: 4 **Cooking Time:** 15 minutes

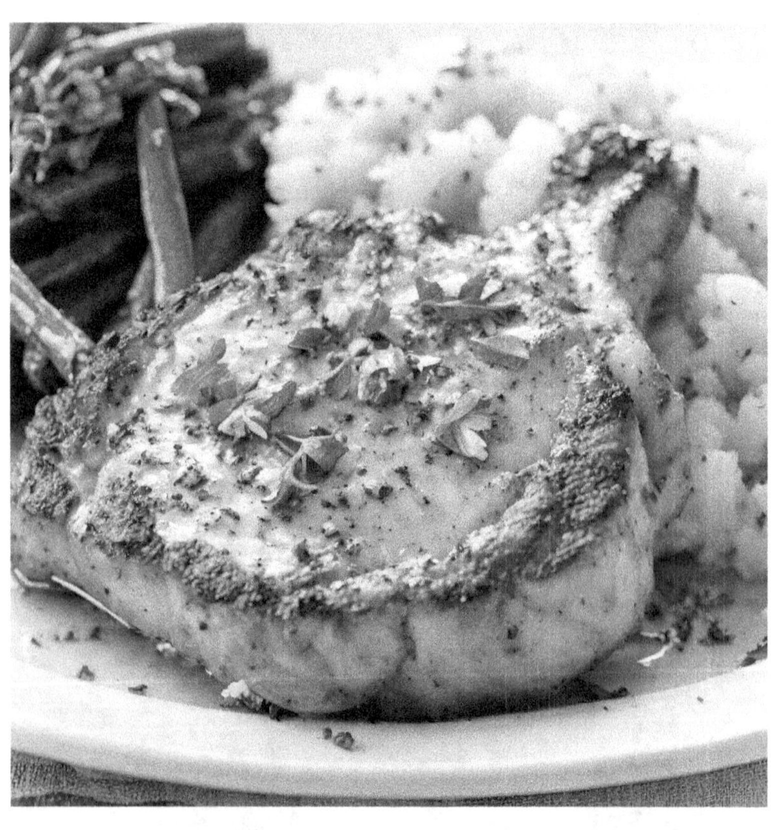

14. Moroccan Spiced Meatballs

Ingredients:

- 1 pound ground beef
- 1 onion, finely chopped
- 2 cloves garlic, minced
- 1 teaspoon cumin
- 1 teaspoon paprika
- 1/2 teaspoon cinnamon
- 1/4 teaspoon cayenne pepper
- Salt and pepper, to taste
- 2 tablespoons olive oil
- 1/2 cup tomato sauce

Instructions:

1. In a bowl, mix together ground beef, onion, garlic, cumin, paprika, cinnamon, cayenne, salt, and pepper. Form into small meatballs.
2. Heat olive oil in a skillet over medium heat. Add meatballs and cook until browned on all sides.
3. Pour tomato sauce over the meatballs and simmer for about 10 minutes, until the sauce is thickened and the meatballs are cooked through.
4. Serve hot, garnished with fresh cilantro if desired.

Nutrition Info Per Serving:

- Calories: 330
- Fat: 20g
- Carbohydrates: 8g
- Protein: 28g
- Fiber: 1g

Serves: 4 **Cooking Time:** 30 minutes

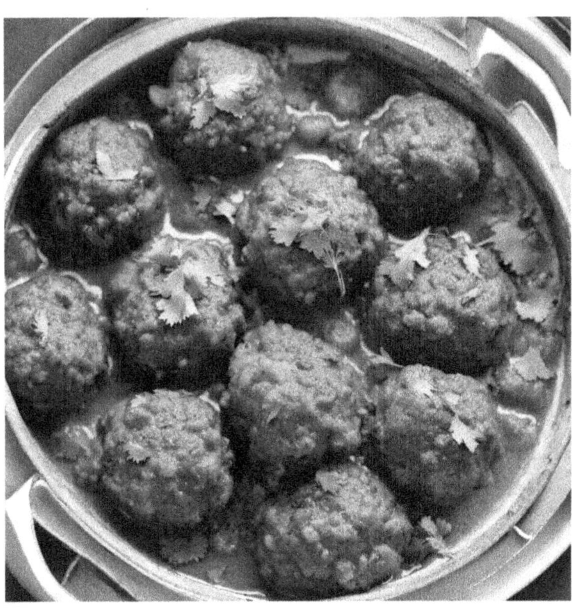

15. Italian Herbed Steak

Ingredients:

- 4 ribeye steaks (about 8 oz each)
- 2 tablespoons olive oil
- 1 tablespoon Italian seasoning
- 2 cloves garlic, minced
- Salt and pepper, to taste

Instructions:

1. Preheat a grill or skillet over medium-high heat.
2. Rub each steak with olive oil and then sprinkle with Italian seasoning, garlic, salt, and pepper.
3. Grill the steaks for about 4-5 minutes per side for medium-rare, adjusting the time depending on your preferred doneness.
4. Let the steaks rest for a few minutes before serving.

Nutrition Info Per Serving:

- Calories: 550
- Fat: 42g
- Carbohydrates: 1g
- Protein: 40g
- Fiber: 0g

Serves: 4 Cooking Time: 10 minutes

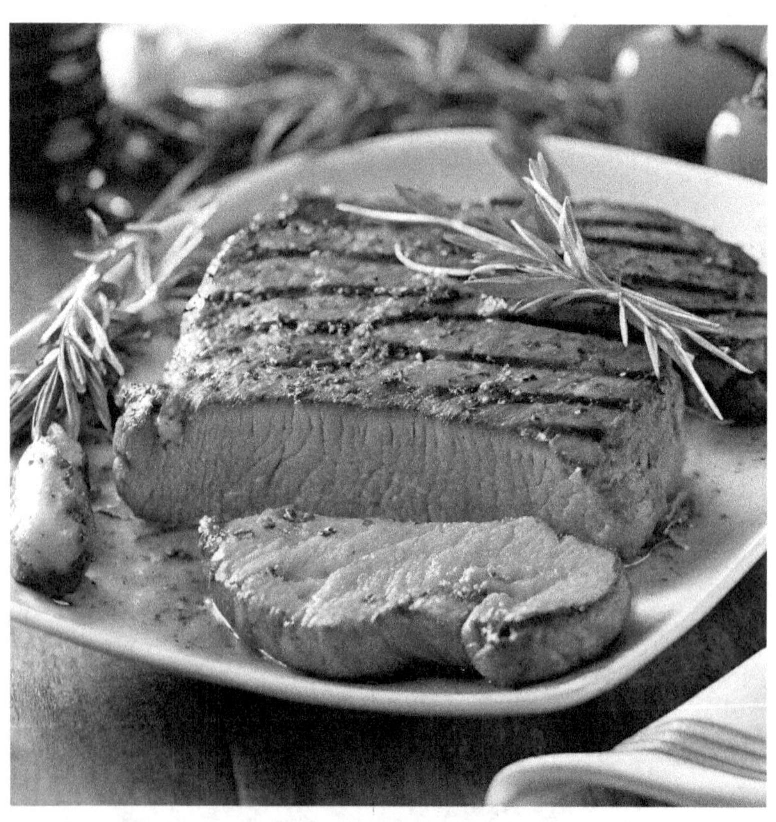

16. Meatloaf Muffins

Ingredients:

- 1 pound ground beef
- 1/2 cup breadcrumbs
- 1/4 cup ketchup
- 1 egg, beaten
- 1 onion, finely chopped
- 1 teaspoon garlic powder
- 1 teaspoon Worcestershire sauce
- Salt and pepper, to taste

Instructions:

1. Preheat your oven to 375°F (190°C).
2. In a bowl, combine all ingredients and mix well.
3. Grease a muffin tin and divide the mixture into the muffin cups.
4. Bake for 20-25 minutes, or until the meatloaf muffins are cooked through.
5. Serve hot.

Nutrition Info Per Serving:

- Calories: 290
- Fat: 15g
- Carbohydrates: 15g
- Protein: 25g
- Fiber: 1g

Serves: 6 (one muffin each) **Cooking Time:** 30 minutes

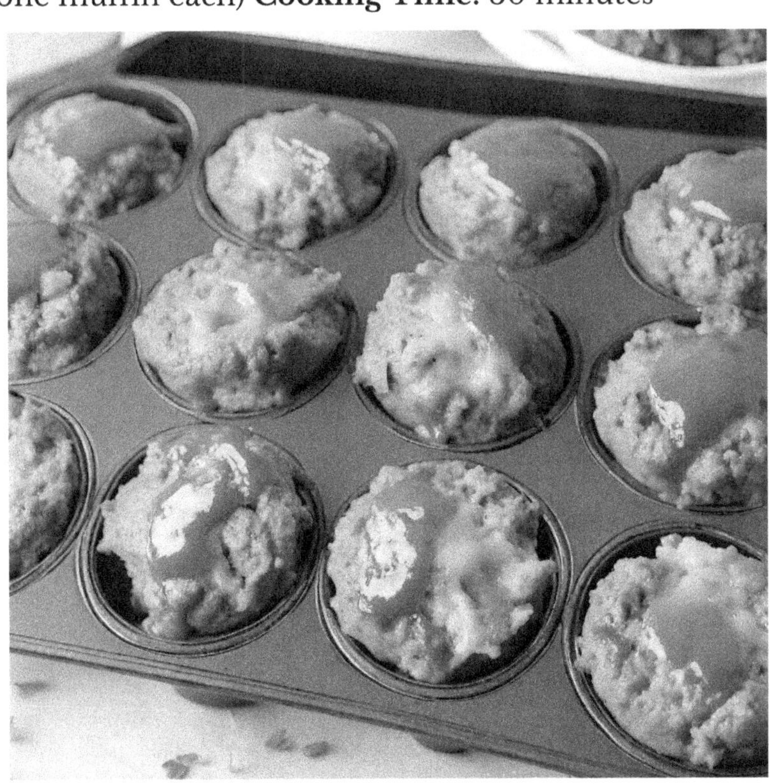

17. Spicy Ground Lamb with Peas

Ingredients:
- 1 pound ground lamb
- 1 cup peas
- 1 onion, diced
- 2 cloves garlic, minced
- 1 tablespoon curry powder
- 1 teaspoon chili powder
- 1/2 cup tomato sauce
- Salt and pepper, to taste
- 2 tablespoons vegetable oil

Instructions:
1. Heat oil in a skillet over medium heat. Add onion and garlic, and sauté until soft.
2. Add ground lamb, curry powder, and chili powder. Cook until lamb is browned.
3. Stir in peas and tomato sauce. Season with salt and pepper.
4. Cook for another 5-10 minutes until everything is heated through and flavors are blended.
5. Serve hot.

Nutrition Info Per Serving:
- Calories: 390
- Fat: 30g
- Carbohydrates: 10g
- Protein: 20g
- Fiber: 3g

Serves: 4 **Cooking Time:** 20 minutes

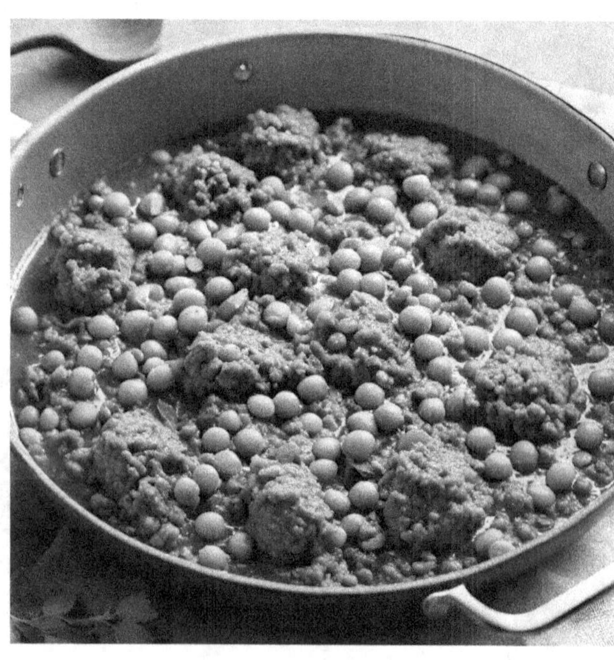

18. Chicken and Beef Kabobs

Ingredients:

- 1/2 pound chicken breast, cubed
- 1/2 pound beef sirloin, cubed
- 2 bell peppers, cut into pieces
- 1 onion, cut into pieces
- Marinade:
    - 1/4 cup olive oil
    - 2 tablespoons soy sauce
    - 1 tablespoon honey
    - 1 clove garlic, minced
    - 1 teaspoon paprika

Instructions:

1. In a bowl, whisk together marinade ingredients.
2. Add chicken and beef cubes to the marinade and let sit for at least 15 minutes.
3. Thread meat and vegetables onto skewers.
4. Preheat grill or broiler. Cook kabobs, turning occasionally, until meat is cooked through and vegetables are tender, about 10-15 minutes.
5. Serve hot.

Nutrition Info Per Serving:

- Calories: 300
- Fat: 16g
- Carbohydrates: 10g
- Protein: 30g
- Fiber: 2g

Serves: 4 **Cooking Time:** 25 minutes

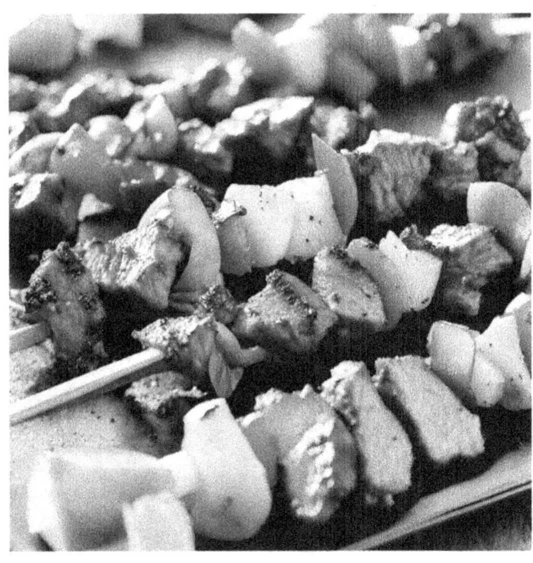

19. Herb-Roasted Turkey Breast

Ingredients:

- 2 pounds turkey breast
- 2 tablespoons olive oil
- 1 tablespoon rosemary, minced
- 1 tablespoon thyme, minced
- Salt and pepper, to taste

Instructions:

1. Preheat oven to 375°F (190°C).
2. Rub turkey breast with olive oil and sprinkle with rosemary, thyme, salt, and pepper.
3. Place in a roasting pan and bake for 25-30 minutes, or until the turkey reaches an internal temperature of 165°F (74°C).
4. Let rest before slicing and serving.

Nutrition Info Per Serving:

- Calories: 165
- Fat: 5g
- Carbohydrates: 0g
- Protein: 30g
- Fiber: 0g

Serves: 4 **Cooking Time:** 30 minutes

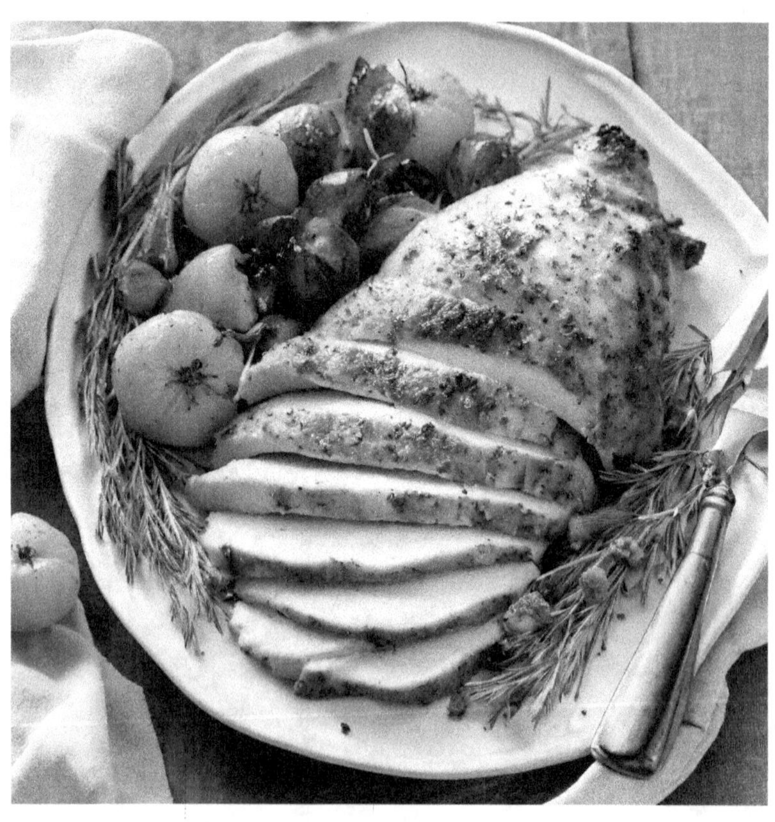

20. Mediterranean Lamb Salad

Ingredients:

- 1 pound lamb shoulder, cooked and sliced
- 4 cups mixed greens
- 1 cup cherry tomatoes, halved
- 1 cucumber, sliced
- 1/2 red onion, thinly sliced
- 1/4 cup feta cheese, crumbled
- 1/4 cup olives, sliced
- Dressing:
  - 1/4 cup olive oil
  - 2 tablespoons red wine vinegar
  - 1 teaspoon Dijon mustard
  - Salt and pepper, to taste

Instructions:

1. In a large salad bowl, combine mixed greens, cherry tomatoes, cucumber, red onion, feta cheese, and olives.
2. Top with sliced lamb.
3. In a small bowl, whisk together olive oil, red wine vinegar, Dijon mustard, salt, and pepper to make the dressing.
4. Drizzle the dressing over the salad and toss to combine.
5. Serve immediately.

Nutrition Info Per Serving:

- Calories: 360
- Fat: 26g
- Carbohydrates: 8g
- Protein: 22g
- Fiber: 2g

Serves: 4 **Cooking Time:** 15 minutes (assuming lamb is pre-cooked)

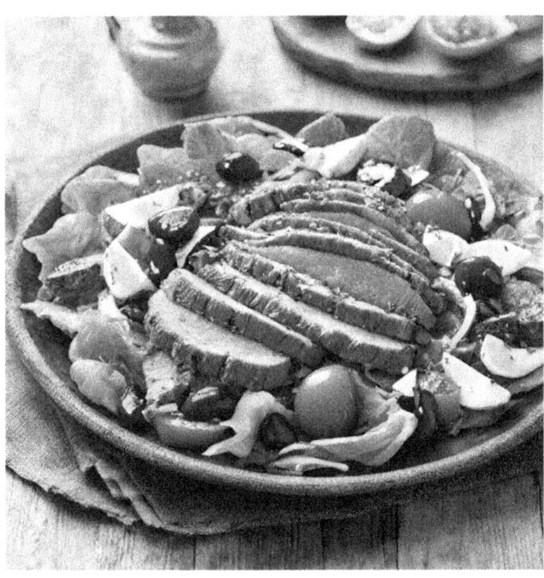

21. Pan-Seared Duck Breast

Ingredients:

- 2 duck breasts, skin on
- Salt and pepper, to taste
- 1 tablespoon olive oil

Instructions:

1. Score the skin of the duck breasts in a criss-cross pattern and season both sides with salt and pepper.
2. Heat olive oil in a skillet over medium heat.
3. Place the duck breasts skin side down in the skillet and cook for about 8 minutes until the skin is crisp and golden.
4. Flip the breasts over and cook for another 4-5 minutes for medium rare.
5. Let rest for 5 minutes, then slice thinly to serve.

Nutrition Info Per Serving:

- Calories: 320
- Fat: 22g
- Carbohydrates: 0g
- Protein: 29g
- Fiber: 0g

Serves: 2 Cooking Time: 20 minutes

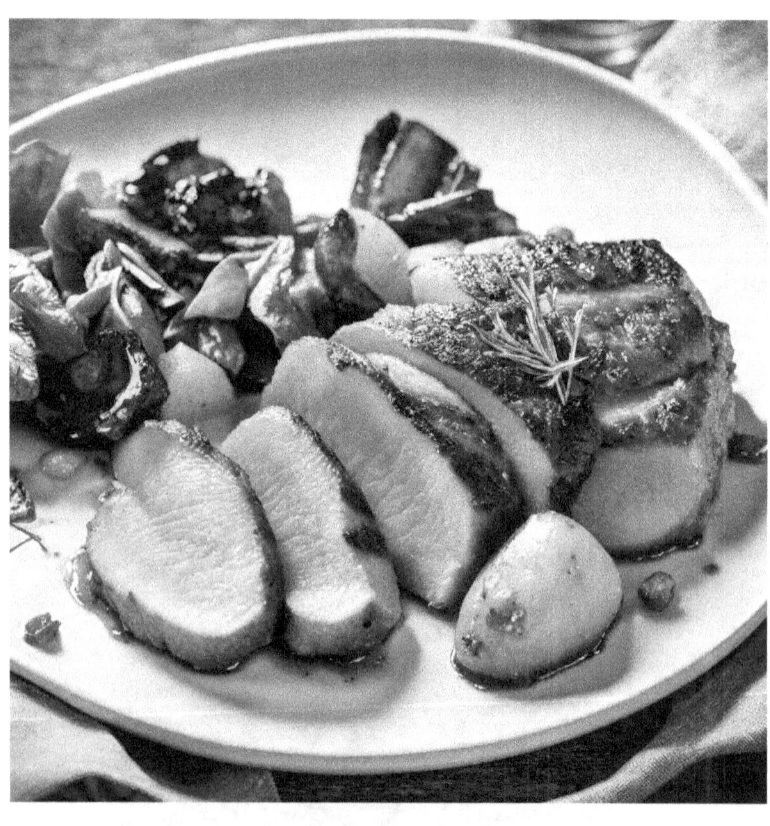

22. Prosciutto-Wrapped Chicken

Ingredients:

- 4 chicken breasts, boneless and skinless
- 8 slices prosciutto
- 1 tablespoon olive oil
- Salt and pepper, to taste
- Fresh herbs for garnish (optional)

Instructions:

1. Preheat your oven to 375°F (190°C).
2. Season chicken breasts with salt and pepper.
3. Wrap each breast with 2 slices of prosciutto, covering as much of the surface as possible.
4. Heat olive oil in an oven-proof skillet over medium-high heat.
5. Sear the chicken on each side for 3 minutes until prosciutto is crispy.
6. Transfer the skillet to the oven and bake for about 10 minutes, until chicken is cooked through.
7. Garnish with fresh herbs before serving.

Nutrition Info Per Serving:

- Calories: 290
- Fat: 14g
- Carbohydrates: 0g
- Protein: 38g
- Fiber: 0g

Serves: 4 **Cooking Time:** 20 minutes

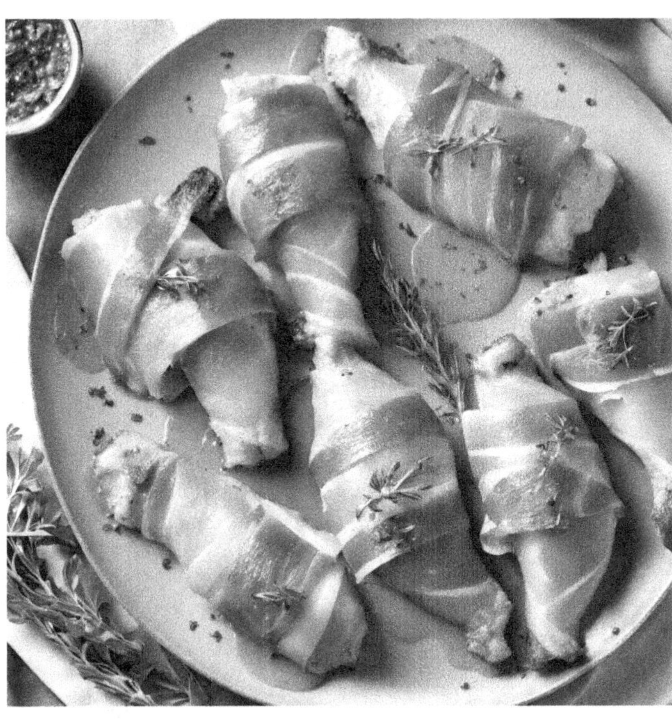

23. Pork and Pineapple Stir-Fry
Ingredients:

- 1 pound pork tenderloin, thinly sliced
- 1 cup pineapple chunks
- 1 bell pepper, sliced
- 1 onion, sliced
- 2 tablespoons soy sauce
- 1 tablespoon honey
- 2 cloves garlic, minced
- 1 tablespoon ginger, minced
- 2 tablespoons vegetable oil

Instructions:

1. Heat 1 tablespoon oil in a large skillet over medium-high heat.
2. Add pork and stir-fry until just cooked, about 3-4 minutes. Remove pork from skillet and set aside.
3. Add remaining oil, garlic, ginger, bell pepper, and onion to the skillet; stir-fry for 2 minutes.
4. Add pineapple and return the pork to the skillet.
5. Whisk together soy sauce and honey, then pour over the stir-fry. Cook for another 2 minutes, stirring frequently.
6. Serve hot.

Nutrition Info Per Serving:

- Calories: 270
- Fat: 12g
- Carbohydrates: 15g
- Protein: 25g
- Fiber: 2g

Serves: 4 Cooking Time: 20 minutes

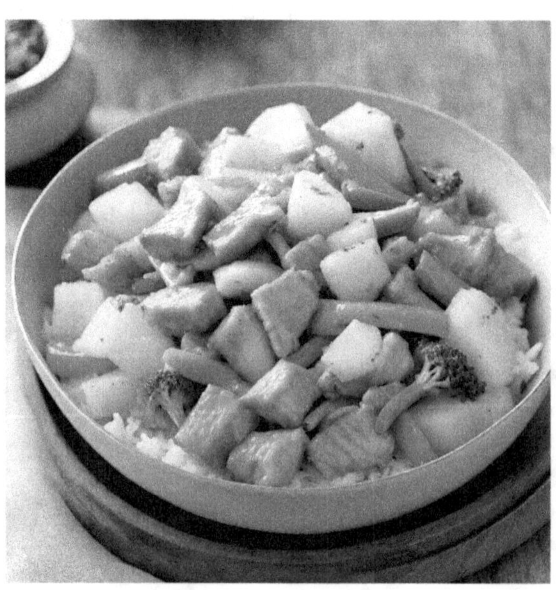

24. Chicken Piccata

Ingredients:

- 4 chicken breast halves, pounded thin
- 1/4 cup flour
- Salt and pepper, to taste
- 4 tablespoons olive oil
- 1/4 cup lemon juice
- 1/2 cup chicken broth
- 1/4 cup capers
- 2 tablespoons parsley, chopped

Instructions:

1. Season the flour with salt and pepper and dredge the chicken breasts in the flour mixture.
2. Heat 2 tablespoons olive oil in a skillet over medium-high heat. Cook the chicken until golden on both sides, about 3-4 minutes per side. Remove chicken from skillet.
3. Add lemon juice, chicken broth, and capers to the skillet. Bring to a simmer.
4. Return the chicken to the skillet and simmer for 5 minutes.
5. Stir in remaining olive oil and sprinkle with parsley before serving.

Nutrition Info Per Serving:

- Calories: 290
- Fat: 15g
- Carbohydrates: 8g
- Protein: 28g
- Fiber: 0.5g

Serves: 4 **Cooking Time:** 20 minutes

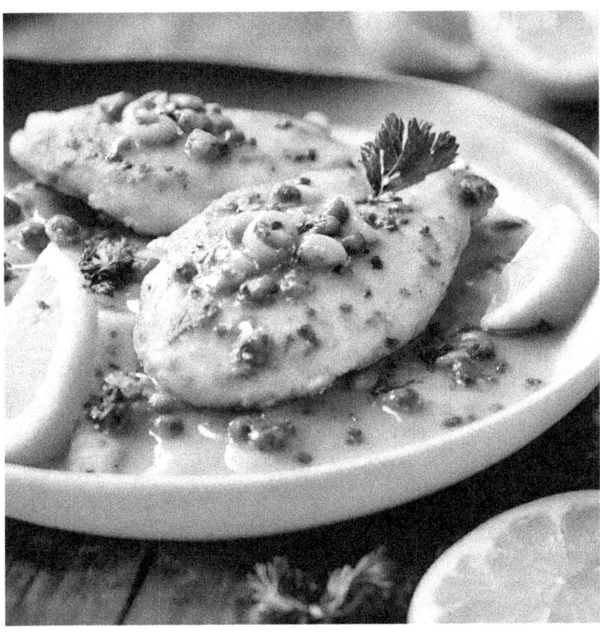

Fish & Seafood Recipes

1. Lemon Garlic Tilapia

Ingredients:

- 4 tilapia fillets (about 6 ounces each)
- 3 tablespoons olive oil
- Juice of 1 lemon
- 3 cloves garlic, minced
- 1 teaspoon dried parsley
- Salt and pepper, to taste
- Lemon slices, for garnish

Instructions:

1. Preheat your oven to 400°F (200°C).
2. In a small bowl, mix together olive oil, lemon juice, minced garlic, parsley, salt, and pepper.
3. Place tilapia fillets in a baking dish and pour the lemon garlic mixture over them.
4. Bake in the preheated oven for about 12-15 minutes, or until the fish flakes easily with a fork.
5. Serve hot, garnished with lemon slices.

Nutrition Info Per Serving:

- Calories: 230
- Fat: 14g
- Carbohydrates: 2g
- Protein: 23g
- Fiber: 0g

Serves: 4 **Cooking Time:** 15 minutes

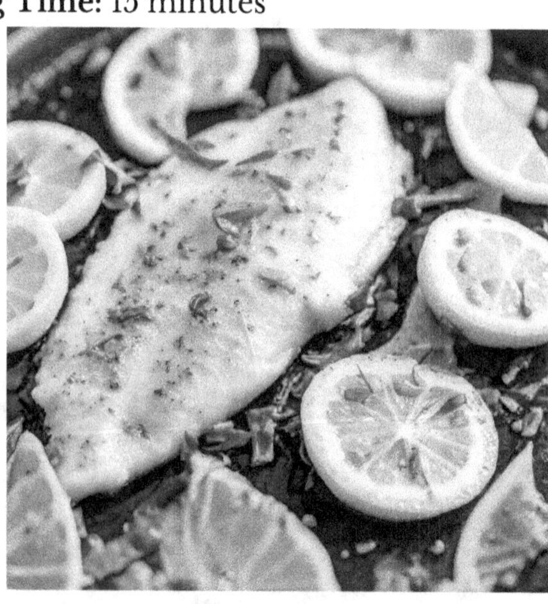

2. Herb-Crusted Salmon

Ingredients:

- 4 salmon fillets (about 6 ounces each)
- 2 tablespoons Dijon mustard
- 2 tablespoons olive oil
- 1/2 cup breadcrumbs
- 1 tablespoon chopped fresh parsley
- 1 teaspoon chopped fresh dill
- Salt and pepper, to taste

Instructions:

1. Preheat your oven to 425°F (220°C).
2. Mix Dijon mustard and olive oil, and brush over the tops of the salmon fillets.
3. In a small bowl, combine breadcrumbs, parsley, dill, salt, and pepper.
4. Press the breadcrumb mixture onto the mustard-coated salmon fillets.
5. Place fillets on a greased baking sheet, and bake for 12-15 minutes, or until the crust is golden and salmon is cooked through.
6. Serve hot.

Nutrition Info Per Serving:

- Calories: 330
- Fat: 18g
- Carbohydrates: 9g
- Protein: 30g
- Fiber: 1g

Serves: 4 **Cooking Time:** 15 minutes

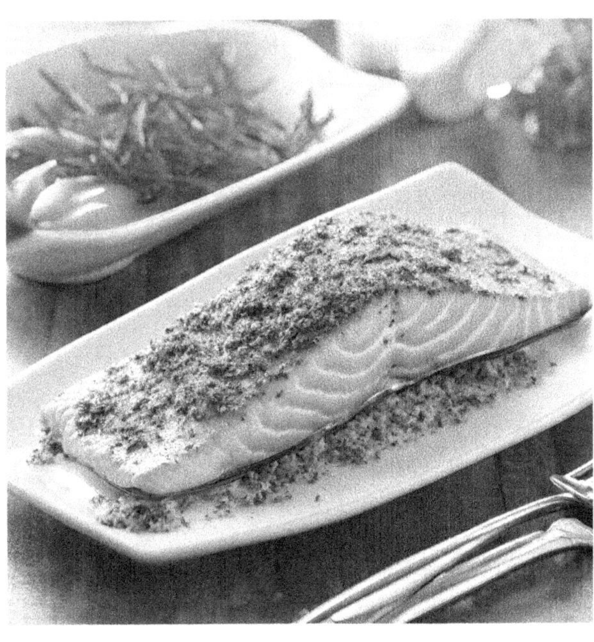

3. Garlic Butter Shrimp
Ingredients:
- 1 pound large shrimp, peeled and deveined
- 4 tablespoons butter
- 4 cloves garlic, minced
- Juice of 1 lemon
- 2 tablespoons chopped fresh parsley
- Salt and pepper, to taste

Instructions:
1. Heat butter in a large skillet over medium heat.
2. Add garlic and sauté for about 1 minute until fragrant.
3. Add shrimp to the skillet, and cook for about 2-3 minutes on each side until pink and cooked through.
4. Stir in lemon juice and parsley, and season with salt and pepper.
5. Serve hot.

Nutrition Info Per Serving:
- Calories: 240
- Fat: 15g
- Carbohydrates: 3g
- Protein: 23g
- Fiber: 0g

Serves: 4 **Cooking Time:** 10 minutes

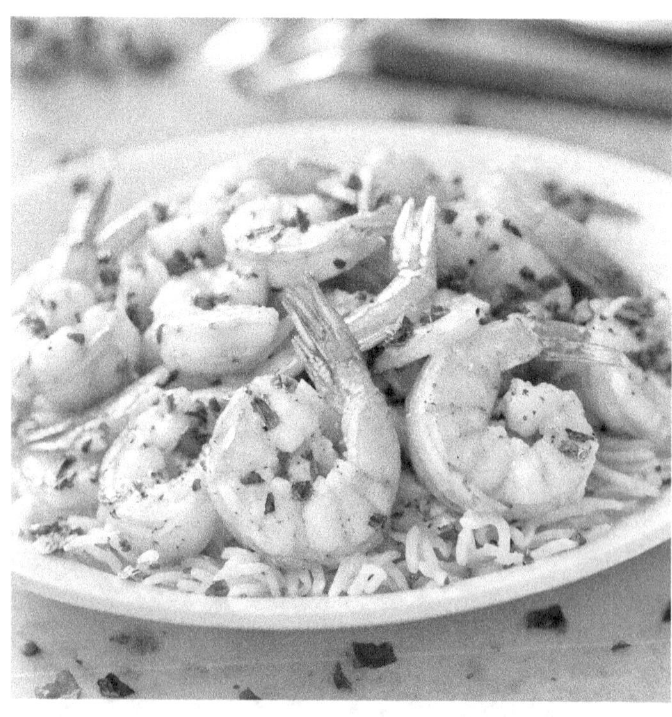

4. Honey Mustard Cod

Ingredients:

- 4 cod fillets (about 6 ounces each)
- 2 tablespoons honey
- 2 tablespoons Dijon mustard
- 1 tablespoon olive oil
- 1 teaspoon apple cider vinegar
- Salt and pepper, to taste
- Lemon wedges, for serving

Instructions:

1. Preheat your oven to 400°F (200°C).
2. In a small bowl, whisk together honey, Dijon mustard, olive oil, apple cider vinegar, salt, and pepper.
3. Place cod fillets in a baking dish and brush each with the honey mustard mixture.
4. Bake for about 12-15 minutes, or until the fish flakes easily with a fork.
5. Serve hot, accompanied by lemon wedges.

Nutrition Info Per Serving:

- Calories: 220
- Fat: 7g
- Carbohydrates: 8g
- Protein: 28g
- Fiber: 0g

Serves: 4 **Cooking Time:** 15 minutes

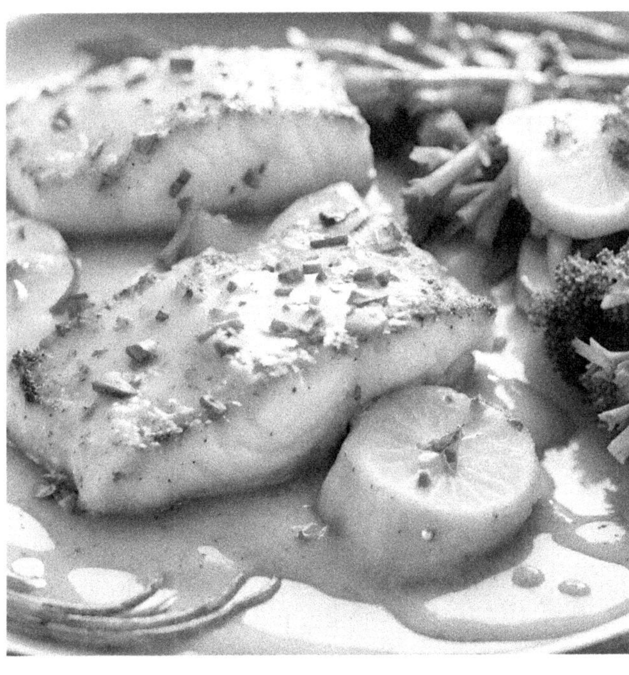

5. Mediterranean Sardine Salad

Ingredients:

- 2 cans sardines in olive oil, drained
- 4 cups mixed salad greens
- 1 cup cherry tomatoes, halved
- 1/2 cucumber, sliced
- 1/4 red onion, thinly sliced
- 1/4 cup olives, halved
- 2 tablespoons capers
- Dressing:
    - 3 tablespoons olive oil
    - 1 tablespoon balsamic vinegar
    - 1 teaspoon Dijon mustard
    - Salt and pepper, to taste

Instructions:

1. In a large salad bowl, combine mixed greens, cherry tomatoes, cucumber, red onion, olives, and capers.
2. Top with sardines.
3. In a small bowl, whisk together olive oil, balsamic vinegar, Dijon mustard, salt, and pepper to make the dressing.
4. Drizzle the dressing over the salad and toss gently to combine.
5. Serve immediately.

Nutrition Info Per Serving:

- Calories: 250
- Fat: 18g
- Carbohydrates: 6g
- Protein: 16g
- Fiber: 2g

Serves: 4 **Cooking Time:** 10 minutes

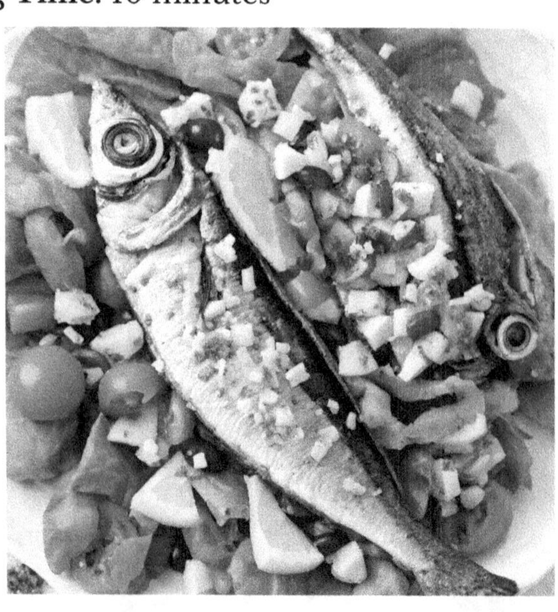

6. Pesto Shrimp Skewers

Ingredients:

- 1 pound large shrimp, peeled and deveined
- 1/4 cup pesto sauce
- 1 tablespoon olive oil
- Lemon wedges, for serving

Instructions:

1. Preheat grill to medium-high heat.
2. Thread shrimp onto skewers.
3. Brush shrimp with olive oil and then coat with pesto sauce.
4. Grill shrimp skewers for 2-3 minutes per side or until shrimp are opaque and cooked through.
5. Serve hot with lemon wedges.

Nutrition Info Per Serving:

- Calories: 210
- Fat: 10g
- Carbohydrates: 2g
- Protein: 25g
- Fiber: 0g

Serves: 4 **Cooking Time:** 10 minutes

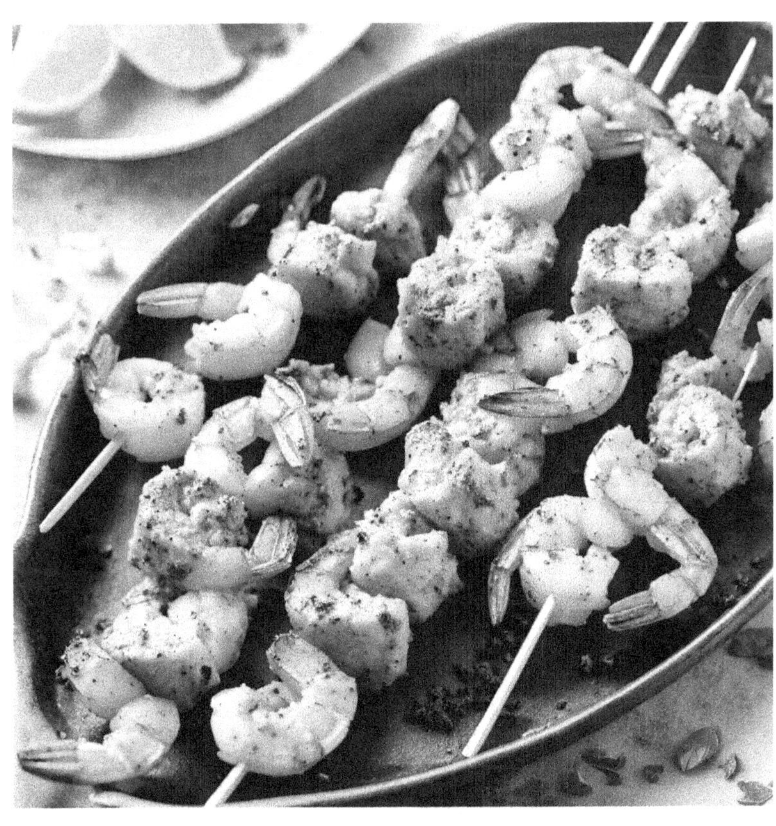

7. Seared Scallops with Lemon Sauce

Ingredients:

- 12 large sea scallops
- 2 tablespoons olive oil
- Salt and pepper, to taste
- Sauce:
  - Juice of 1 lemon
  - 2 tablespoons butter
  - 1 clove garlic, minced
  - 1 tablespoon chopped parsley

Instructions:

1. Pat scallops dry and season with salt and pepper.
2. Heat olive oil in a skillet over high heat.
3. Sear scallops for about 1-2 minutes on each side until a golden crust forms.
4. Remove scallops from skillet and set aside.
5. In the same skillet, add lemon juice, butter, and garlic. Cook for 2 minutes over medium heat, scraping up any browned bits.
6. Stir in parsley and pour sauce over scallops to serve.

Nutrition Info Per Serving:

- Calories: 190
- Fat: 11g
- Carbohydrates: 4g
- Protein: 18g
- Fiber: 0g

Serves: 4 **Cooking Time:** 10 minutes

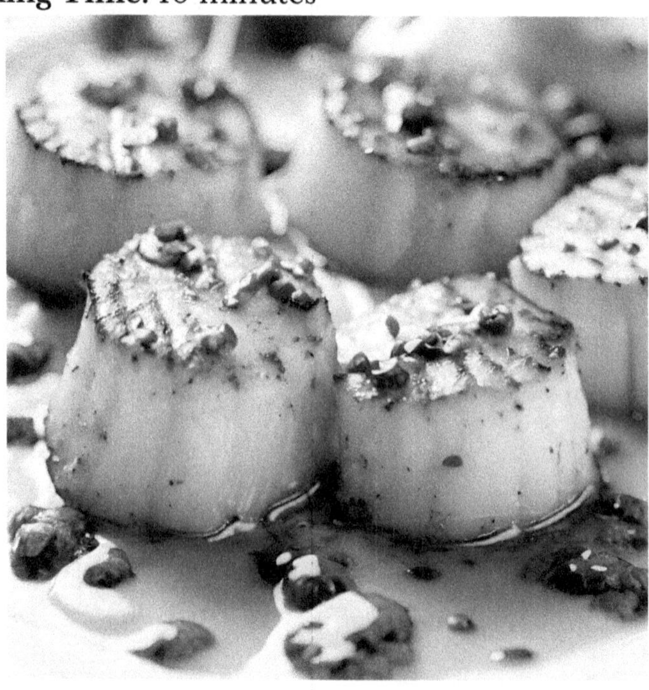

8. Smoked Salmon Breakfast Wrap

Ingredients:

- 4 whole wheat tortillas
- 8 ounces smoked salmon
- 1 avocado, sliced
- 1/2 cup cream cheese
- 1/4 red onion, thinly sliced
- 2 tablespoons capers
- Fresh dill, for garnish

Instructions:

1. Spread each tortilla with cream cheese.
2. Top with smoked salmon, avocado slices, red onion, capers, and fresh dill.
3. Roll up the tortillas tightly, slice in half, and serve.

Nutrition Info Per Serving:

- Calories: 380
- Fat: 22g
- Carbohydrates: 27g
- Protein: 20g
- Fiber: 5g

Serves: 4 **Cooking Time:** 10 minutes

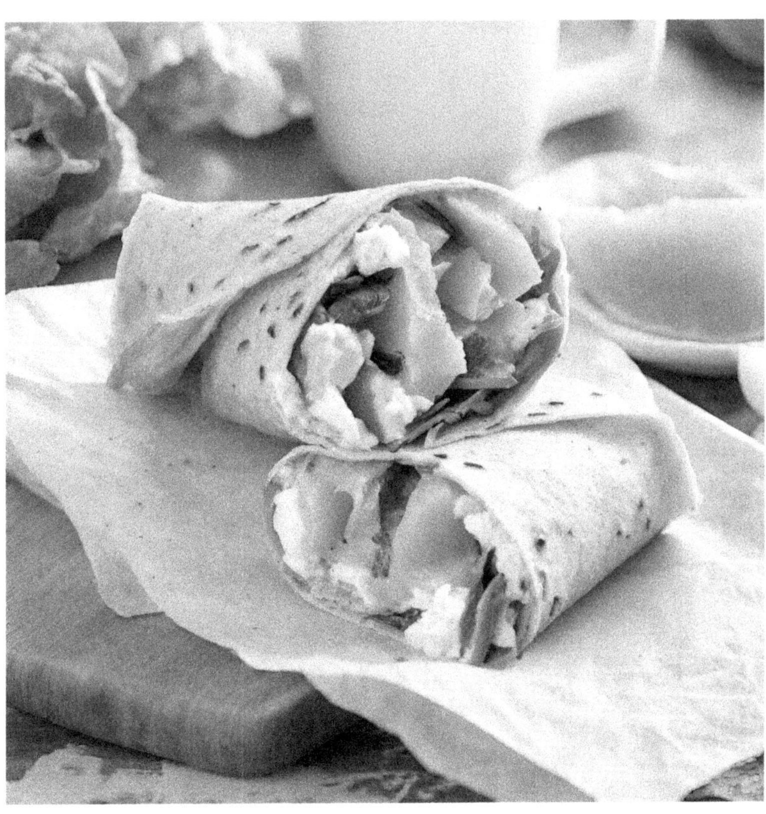

9. Grilled Mackerel with Herbs

Ingredients:

- 4 mackerel fillets
- 2 tablespoons olive oil
- 1 lemon, sliced
- Fresh herbs (such as parsley, thyme, and rosemary), chopped
- Salt and pepper, to taste

Instructions:

1. Preheat grill to medium-high heat.
2. Brush mackerel fillets with olive oil and season with salt and pepper.
3. Place lemon slices and fresh herbs under and on top of the fish.
4. Grill for 4-5 minutes per side, or until fish is cooked through and flakes easily.
5. Serve immediately, garnished with additional herbs if desired.

Nutrition Info Per Serving:

- Calories: 290
- Fat: 20g
- Carbohydrates: 2g
- Protein: 24g
- Fiber: 0.5g

Serves: 4 **Cooking Time:** 10 minutes

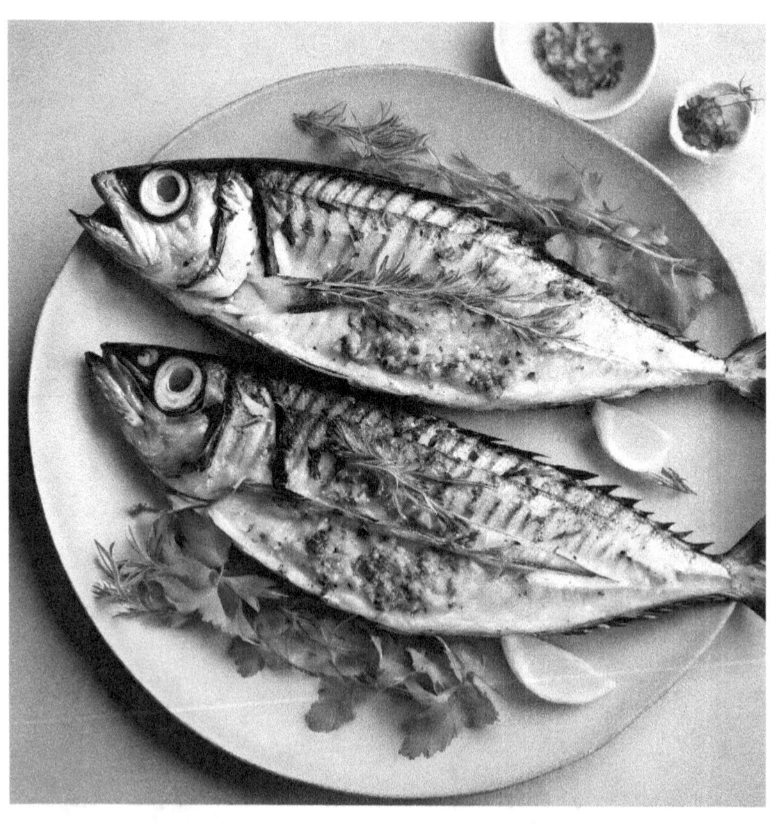

10. Clam Chowder (Dairy-Free)

Ingredients:

- 2 cups canned clams in juice
- 1 onion, chopped
- 2 potatoes, diced
- 2 carrots, diced
- 1 stalk celery, diced
- 4 cups vegetable broth
- 1 cup coconut milk
- 2 tablespoons olive oil
- 1 teaspoon thyme
- Salt and pepper, to taste

Instructions:

1. In a large pot, heat olive oil over medium heat.
2. Add onion, carrots, and celery, and sauté until onions are translucent.
3. Add potatoes, clams with their juice, and vegetable broth.
4. Bring to a boil, then reduce heat and simmer for about 15 minutes, until potatoes are tender.
5. Stir in coconut milk, thyme, salt, and pepper, and heat through.
6. Serve hot.

Nutrition Info Per Serving:

- Calories: 210
- Fat: 10g
- Carbohydrates: 24g
- Protein: 8g
- Fiber: 3g

Serves: 4 **Cooking Time:** 25 minutes

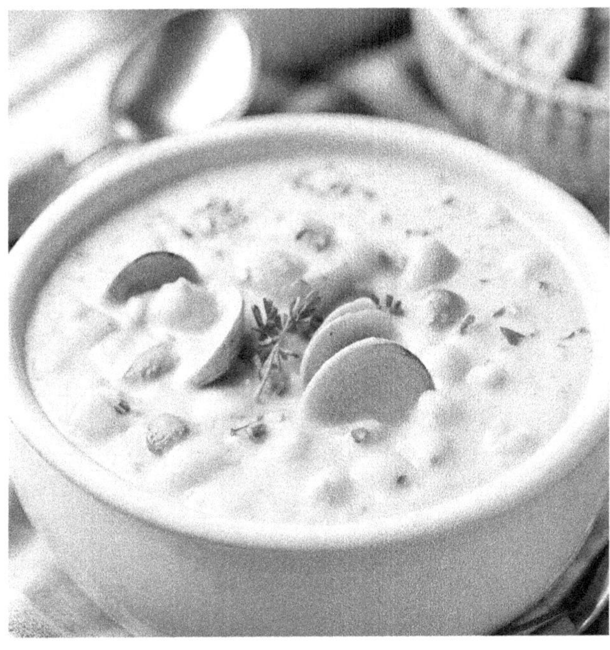

11. Crab Salad with Citrus Vinaigrette

Ingredients:

- 1 pound crab meat, picked over for shells
- 1 avocado, diced
- 1/2 cucumber, diced
- 1/4 red onion, thinly sliced
- 1 orange, segmented
- Dressing:
  - Juice of 1 lemon
  - Juice of 1 orange
  - 2 tablespoons olive oil
  - 1 teaspoon honey
  - Salt and pepper, to taste

Instructions:

1. In a large bowl, combine crab meat, avocado, cucumber, red onion, and orange segments.
2. In a small bowl, whisk together lemon juice, orange juice, olive oil, honey, salt, and pepper.
3. Pour the dressing over the salad and toss gently to coat.
4. Chill for about 10 minutes before serving to allow flavors to meld.

Nutrition Info Per Serving:

- Calories: 290
- Fat: 15g
- Carbohydrates: 20g
- Protein: 20g
- Fiber: 4g

Serves: 4 **Cooking Time:** 20 minutes

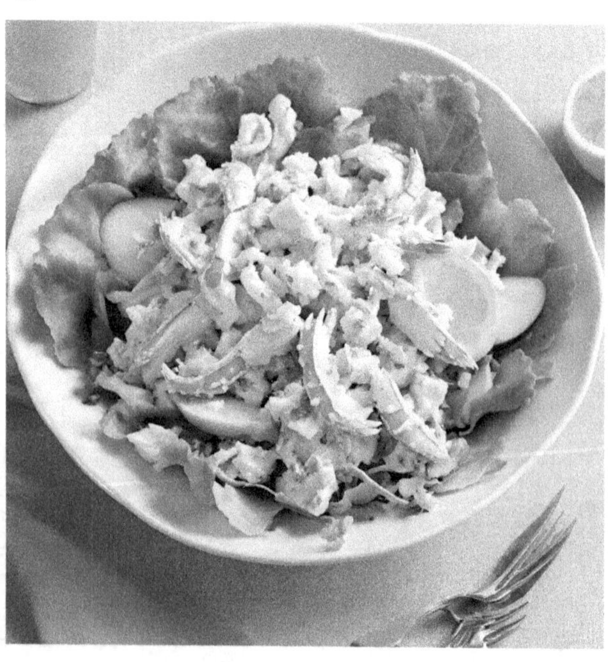

12. Thai Coconut Shrimp Soup
Ingredients:

- 1 pound shrimp, peeled and deveined
- 1 can (14 oz) coconut milk
- 2 cups chicken broth
- 1 tablespoon red curry paste
- 1 stalk lemongrass, minced
- 1 inch piece ginger, grated
- 1 bell pepper, sliced
- 1 cup mushrooms, sliced
- Juice of 1 lime
- 2 tablespoons fish sauce
- 1/4 cup cilantro, chopped
- 1 tablespoon oil

Instructions:

1. Heat oil in a large pot over medium heat. Add ginger, lemongrass, and red curry paste, sauté for 2 minutes.
2. Pour in coconut milk and chicken broth, bring to a simmer.
3. Add bell pepper and mushrooms, cook for 5 minutes.
4. Add shrimp and cook until they turn pink, about 3-5 minutes.
5. Stir in lime juice, fish sauce, and cilantro.
6. Serve hot.

Nutrition Info Per Serving:

- Calories: 320
- Fat: 20g
- Carbohydrates: 8g
- Protein: 25g
- Fiber: 1g

Serves: 4 Cooking Time: 20 minutes

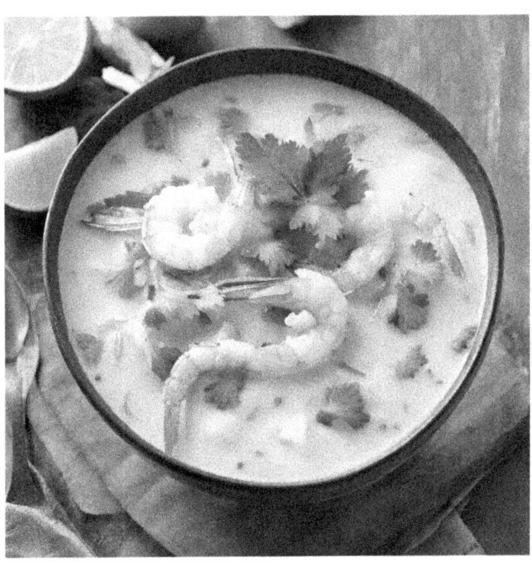

13. Garlic Lemon Mussels

Ingredients:

- 2 pounds mussels, cleaned and de-bearded
- 3 tablespoons butter
- 4 cloves garlic, minced
- Juice of 1 lemon
- 1/4 cup white wine
- 1/4 cup parsley, chopped
- Salt and pepper, to taste

Instructions:

1. In a large pot, melt butter over medium heat. Add garlic and sauté for 1 minute.
2. Pour in lemon juice and white wine, bring to a simmer.
3. Add mussels and cover the pot. Cook for 5-7 minutes until all mussels have opened. Discard any that do not open.
4. Season with salt and pepper, and sprinkle with parsley.
5. Serve hot with crusty bread.

Nutrition Info Per Serving:

- Calories: 300
- Fat: 15g
- Carbohydrates: 10g
- Protein: 25g
- Fiber: 0g

Serves: 4 **Cooking Time:** 15 minutes

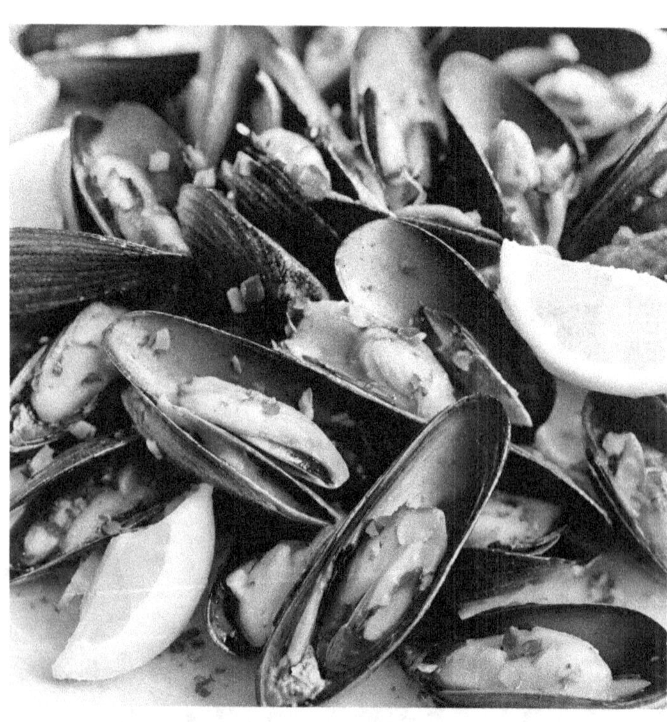

14. Pan-Fried Calamari with Aioli

Ingredients:
- 1 pound calamari rings
- 1/2 cup flour
- 1 teaspoon paprika
- Salt and pepper, to taste
- 1/2 cup olive oil
- For the Aioli:
    - 1/2 cup mayonnaise
    - 1 clove garlic, minced
    - 1 tablespoon lemon juice

Instructions:
1. In a bowl, mix flour, paprika, salt, and pepper.
2. Dredge calamari rings in the flour mixture.
3. Heat oil in a frying pan over medium-high heat. Fry calamari for 2-3 minutes until golden and crispy.
4. Drain on paper towels.
5. For the aioli, mix mayonnaise, garlic, and lemon juice in a small bowl.
6. Serve calamari hot with aioli on the side.

Nutrition Info Per Serving:
- Calories: 450
- Fat: 30g
- Carbohydrates: 18g
- Protein: 25g
- Fiber: 1g

Serves: 4 **Cooking Time:** 15 minutes

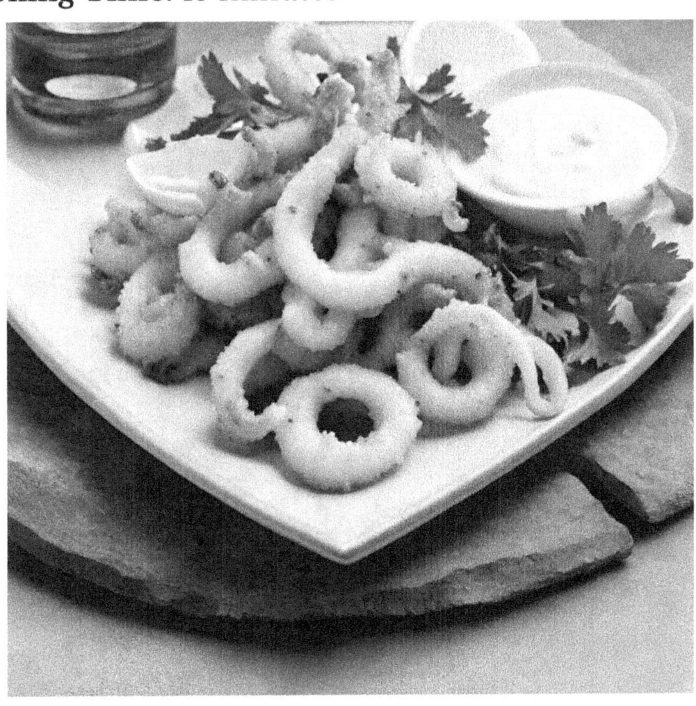

15. Shrimp and Avocado Taco Salad
Ingredients:
- 1 pound cooked shrimp, peeled and deveined
- 4 cups mixed greens
- 1 avocado, diced
- 1 cup cherry tomatoes, halved
- 1/2 cup corn kernels
- 1/4 cup red onion, thinly sliced
- 1/2 cup cilantro, chopped
- 2 tablespoons olive oil
- Juice of 1 lime
- 1 teaspoon chili powder
- Salt and pepper, to taste

Instructions:
1. In a large salad bowl, combine mixed greens, avocado, cherry tomatoes, corn, red onion, and cilantro.
2. In a small bowl, whisk together olive oil, lime juice, chili powder, salt, and pepper.
3. Toss the shrimp in the dressing and then add to the salad.
4. Toss everything together and serve immediately.

Nutrition Info Per Serving:
- Calories: 290
- Fat: 15g
- Carbohydrates: 13g
- Protein: 25g
- Fiber: 5g

Serves: 4 Cooking Time: 10 minutes

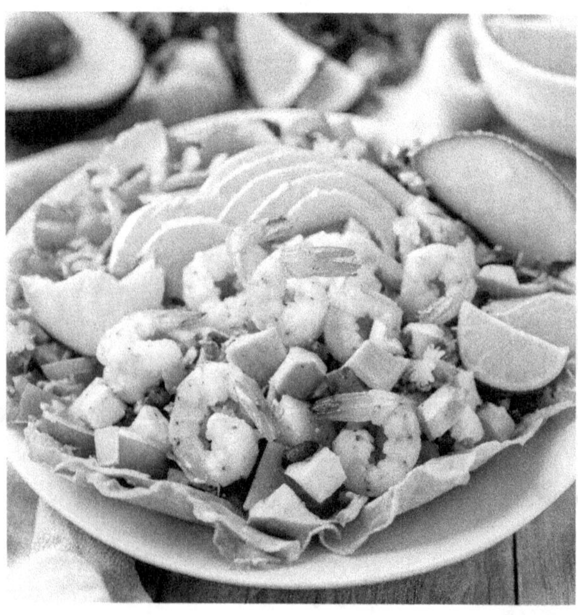

16. Lobster Tail with Herb Butter

Ingredients:

- 4 lobster tails
- 4 tablespoons butter, melted
- 1 tablespoon chopped fresh parsley
- 1 clove garlic, minced
- 1 teaspoon lemon zest
- Salt and pepper, to taste
- Lemon wedges, for serving

Instructions:

1. Preheat your broiler.
2. Split the lobster tails down the middle with a sharp knife or kitchen shears.
3. In a small bowl, mix together melted butter, parsley, garlic, lemon zest, salt, and pepper.
4. Place lobster tails on a baking sheet, and brush generously with the butter mixture.
5. Broil 5-10 minutes, depending on the size of the tails, or until the meat is opaque and cooked through.
6. Serve immediately with lemon wedges on the side.

Nutrition Info Per Serving:

- Calories: 250
- Fat: 15g
- Carbohydrates: 1g
- Protein: 25g
- Fiber: 0g

Serves: 4 **Cooking Time:** 15 minutes

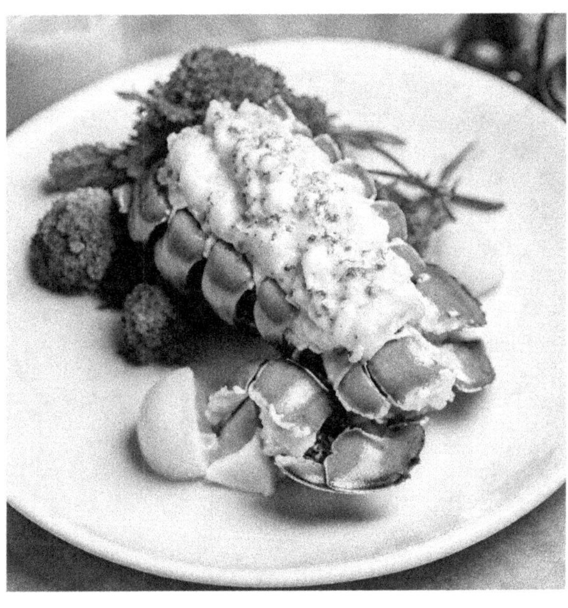

17. Oyster Mushroom Ceviche

Ingredients:

- 2 cups oyster mushrooms, thinly sliced
- 1/2 cup lime juice
- 1/4 cup orange juice
- 1 red onion, finely chopped
- 1 cucumber, peeled and diced
- 1 jalapeño, seeded and finely chopped
- 1/4 cup cilantro, chopped
- Salt and pepper, to taste

Instructions:

1. In a bowl, combine mushrooms with lime and orange juice. Let marinate for 15 minutes in the refrigerator.
2. Add red onion, cucumber, jalapeño, and cilantro to the mushrooms. Season with salt and pepper to taste.
3. Mix well and let sit for another 10 minutes to blend the flavors.
4. Serve chilled as an appetizer or light main dish.

Nutrition Info Per Serving:

- Calories: 60
- Fat: 0.5g
- Carbohydrates: 10g
- Protein: 2g
- Fiber: 2g

Serves: 4 Cooking Time: 25 minutes

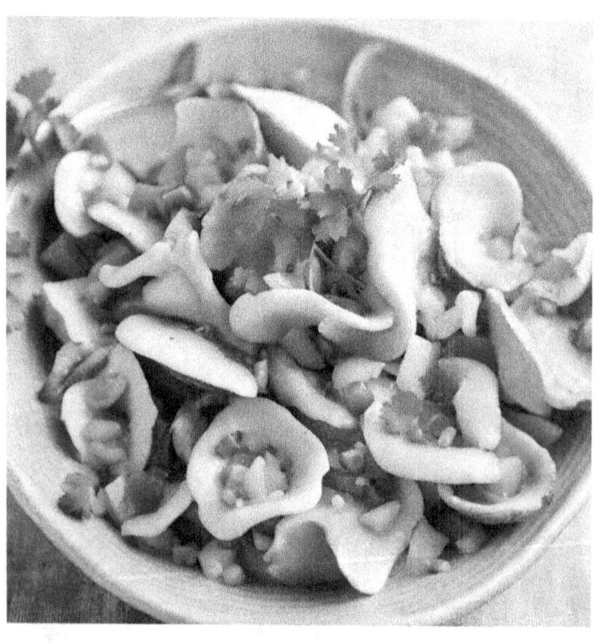

18. Baked Clams with Garlic

Ingredients:

- 24 clams, cleaned
- 4 cloves garlic, minced
- 1/2 cup breadcrumbs
- 1/4 cup parsley, chopped
- 1/4 cup grated Parmesan cheese
- 1/4 cup olive oil
- Lemon wedges, for serving

Instructions:

1. Preheat your oven to 375°F (190°C).
2. In a bowl, mix together garlic, breadcrumbs, parsley, Parmesan cheese, and olive oil.
3. Place clams on a baking sheet. Spoon breadcrumb mixture onto each clam.
4. Bake for 10 minutes, or until the clams are fully opened and the topping is golden.
5. Serve hot with lemon wedges.

Nutrition Info Per Serving:

- Calories: 250
- Fat: 15g
- Carbohydrates: 15g
- Protein: 15g
- Fiber: 1g

Serves: 4 Cooking Time: 20 minutes

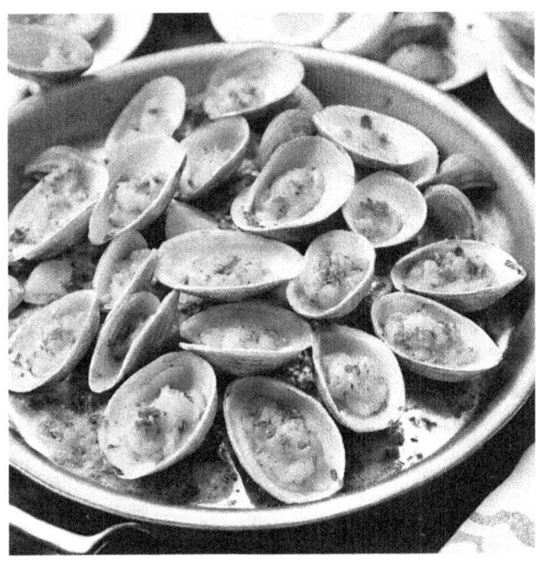

19. Scallops with Asparagus
Ingredients:
- 12 large sea scallops
- 1 bunch asparagus, trimmed
- 2 tablespoons olive oil
- Salt and pepper, to taste
- 1 lemon, juiced

Instructions:
1. Heat olive oil in a large skillet over medium-high heat.
2. Season scallops with salt and pepper. Add to the skillet and sear on each side for about 2 minutes until golden brown.
3. Remove scallops and add asparagus to the skillet. Cook for about 3-5 minutes until tender but still crisp.
4. Return scallops to the skillet, squeeze lemon juice over everything, and cook for an additional minute.
5. Serve immediately.

Nutrition Info Per Serving:
- Calories: 200
- Fat: 10g
- Carbohydrates: 8g
- Protein: 20g
- Fiber: 2g

Serves: 4 Cooking Time: 15 minutes

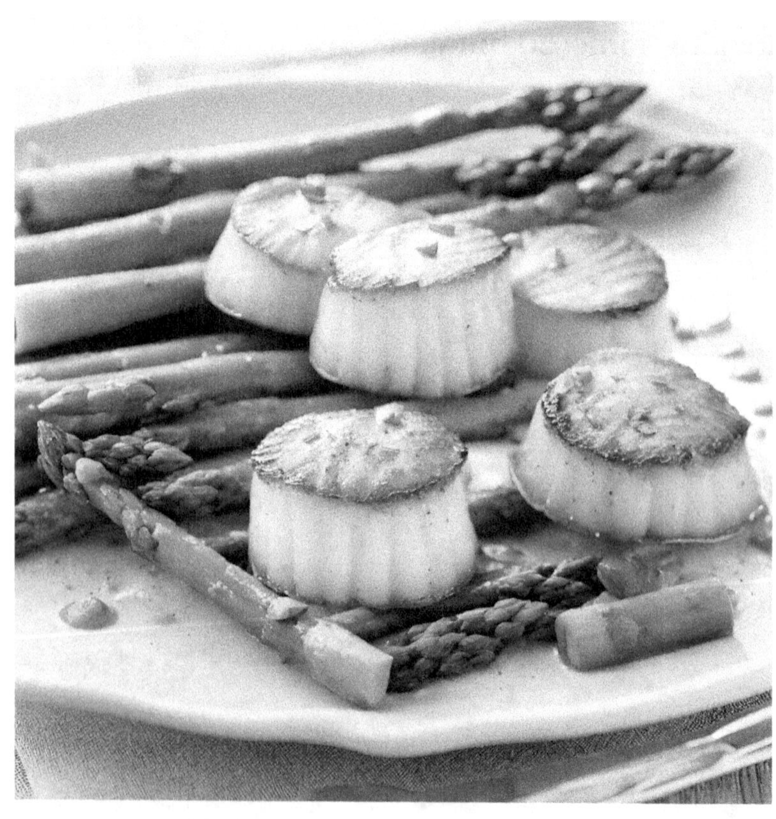

20. Moroccan Grilled Fish

Ingredients:

- 4 fish fillets (such as cod or tilapia)
- 2 tablespoons olive oil
- 2 cloves garlic, minced
- 1 teaspoon paprika
- 1 teaspoon cumin
- 1/2 teaspoon coriander
- 1/4 teaspoon cayenne pepper
- Juice of 1 lemon
- Salt and pepper, to taste
- Fresh cilantro, for garnish

Instructions:

1. In a small bowl, mix together olive oil, garlic, paprika, cumin, coriander, cayenne, lemon juice, salt, and pepper.
2. Rub the marinade over the fish fillets and let sit for 10 minutes.
3. Preheat grill to medium-high heat and oil the grates.
4. Grill the fish for about 4-5 minutes on each side, or until cooked through and easily flakes with a fork.
5. Garnish with fresh cilantro and serve.

Nutrition Info Per Serving:

- Calories: 220
- Fat: 10g
- Carbohydrates: 2g
- Protein: 30g
- Fiber: 0g

Serves: 4 **Cooking Time:** 20 minutes

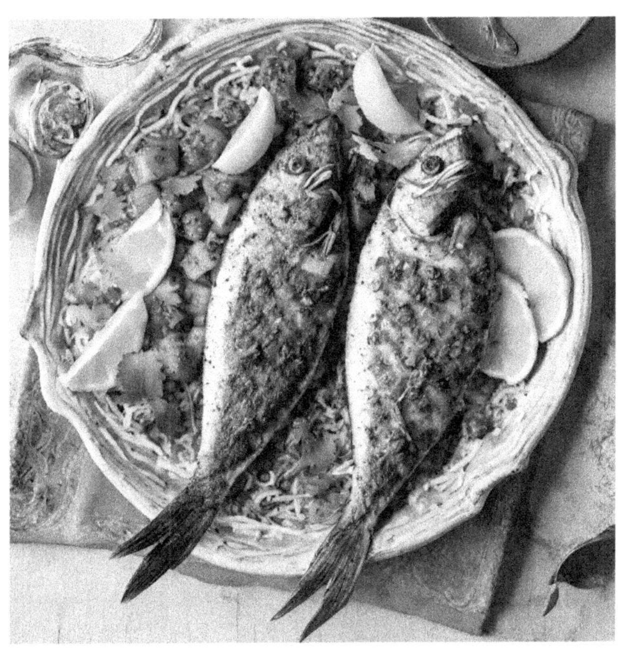

21. Asian-Style Tuna Steaks

Ingredients:

- 4 tuna steaks (about 6 ounces each)
- 1/4 cup soy sauce
- 2 tablespoons sesame oil
- 1 tablespoon honey
- 1 clove garlic, minced
- 1 teaspoon grated ginger
- 1 tablespoon sesame seeds
- Green onions, sliced for garnish

Instructions:

1. In a small bowl, whisk together soy sauce, sesame oil, honey, garlic, and ginger.
2. Place tuna steaks in a dish and pour the marinade over them. Let marinate for 15 minutes.
3. Heat a grill pan over high heat. Remove tuna from marinade and sear for 2-3 minutes on each side for medium-rare.
4. Sprinkle with sesame seeds and sliced green onions before serving.

Nutrition Info Per Serving:

- Calories: 290
- Fat: 14g
- Carbohydrates: 5g
- Protein: 35g
- Fiber: 0g

Serves: 4 **Cooking Time:** 20 minutes

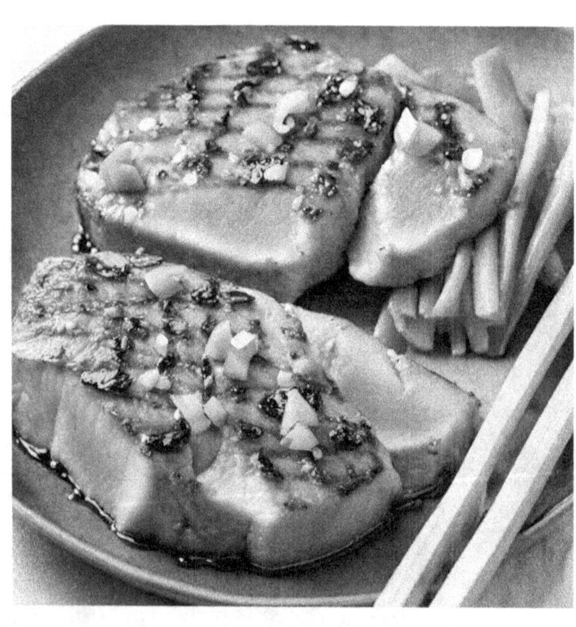

22. Indian-Spiced Shrimp Curry

Ingredients:

- 1 pound shrimp, peeled and deveined
- 1 tablespoon vegetable oil
- 1 onion, finely chopped
- 2 cloves garlic, minced
- 1 tablespoon grated ginger
- 1 tablespoon curry powder
- 1 can (14 oz) coconut milk
- 1 tomato, diced
- Fresh cilantro, for garnish
- Salt and pepper, to taste

Instructions:

1. Heat oil in a skillet over medium heat. Add onion, garlic, and ginger, and sauté until onion is translucent.
2. Stir in curry powder and cook for 1 minute until fragrant.
3. Add coconut milk and bring to a simmer.
4. Add shrimp and tomato, and cook until shrimp are pink and cooked through, about 5 minutes.
5. Season with salt and pepper, garnish with cilantro, and serve.

Nutrition Info Per Serving:

- Calories: 280
- Fat: 18g
- Carbohydrates: 8g
- Protein: 24g
- Fiber: 1g

Serves: 4 **Cooking Time:** 20 minutes

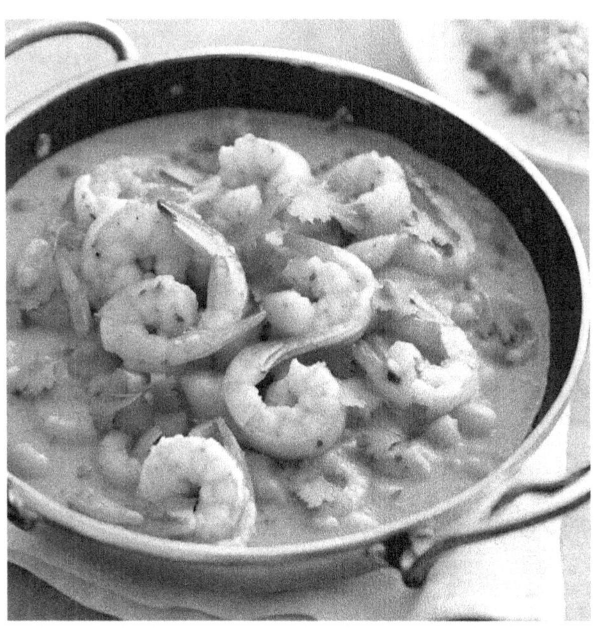

23. Greek-Style Baked Sardines

Ingredients:

- 1 pound fresh sardines, cleaned
- 1/4 cup olive oil
- Juice of 1 lemon
- 3 cloves garlic, sliced
- 1 tablespoon dried oregano
- Salt and pepper, to taste
- Lemon slices and fresh parsley, for garnish

Instructions:

1. Preheat oven to 375°F (190°C).
2. Arrange sardines in a single layer in a baking dish.
3. In a small bowl, mix olive oil, lemon juice, garlic, oregano, salt, and pepper.
4. Pour the mixture over the sardines.
5. Bake for 15-20 minutes, until sardines are cooked through.
6. Garnish with lemon slices and parsley before serving.

Nutrition Info Per Serving:

- Calories: 210
- Fat: 14g
- Carbohydrates: 2g
- Protein: 20g
- Fiber: 0g

Serves: 4 **Cooking Time:** 25 minutes

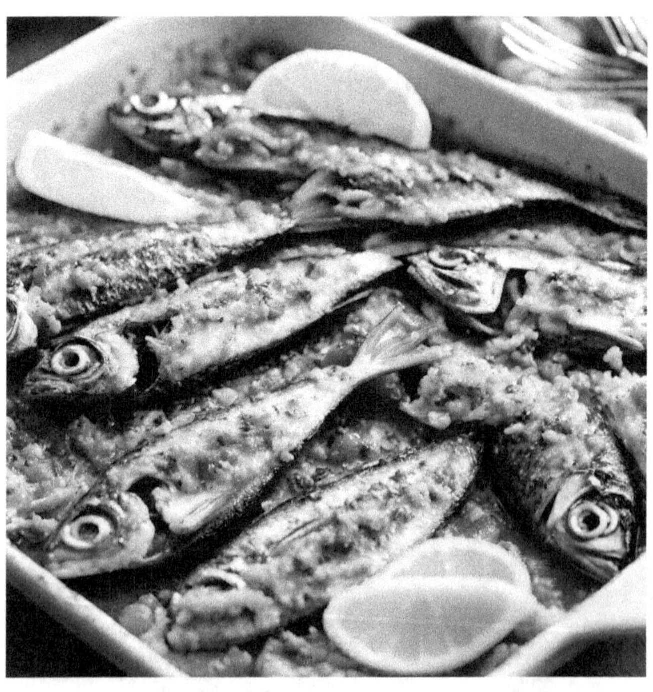

24. Quick Fish Stew

Ingredients:

- 1 pound firm white fish fillets (like cod or halibut), cut into chunks
- 1 tablespoon olive oil
- 1 onion, chopped
- 2 cloves garlic, minced
- 1 bell pepper, chopped
- 1 can (14 oz) diced tomatoes
- 1 cup vegetable broth
- 1 teaspoon paprika
- 1 teaspoon dried thyme
- Salt and pepper, to taste
- Fresh parsley, chopped for garnish

Instructions:

1. Heat olive oil in a large pot over medium heat. Add onion and garlic, and sauté until soft.
2. Add bell pepper, tomatoes, vegetable broth, paprika, and thyme. Bring to a simmer.
3. Add fish chunks to the pot and simmer gently for 10-12 minutes, until fish is cooked through.
4. Season with salt and pepper to taste.
5. Garnish with fresh parsley before serving.

Nutrition Info Per Serving:

- Calories: 220
- Fat: 6g
- Carbohydrates: 10g
- Protein: 30g
- Fiber: 2g

Serves: 4 **Cooking Time:** 20 minutes

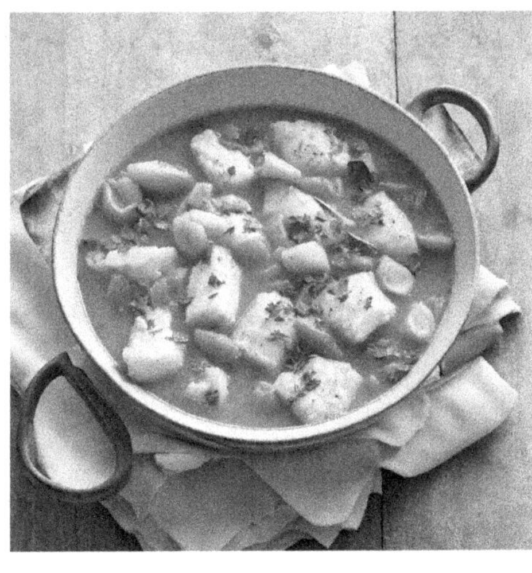

25. Shrimp Alfredo (Dairy-Free)

Ingredients:

- 1 pound shrimp, peeled and deveined
- 1 tablespoon olive oil
- 2 cloves garlic, minced
- 1 cup coconut cream
- 1/4 cup nutritional yeast
- 1 teaspoon Italian seasoning
- Salt and pepper, to taste
- Cooked pasta, for serving
- Fresh parsley, chopped for garnish

Instructions:

1. Heat olive oil in a large skillet over medium heat. Add garlic and sauté until fragrant, about 1 minute.
2. Add shrimp and cook until they are pink and opaque, about 3-4 minutes per side.
3. Lower the heat and stir in coconut cream, nutritional yeast, and Italian seasoning. Simmer for 5 minutes, until the sauce thickens slightly.
4. Season with salt and pepper.
5. Serve the shrimp and sauce over cooked pasta, garnished with chopped parsley.

Nutrition Info Per Serving:

- Calories: 320
- Fat: 20g
- Carbohydrates: 8g
- Protein: 28g
- Fiber: 1g

Serves: 4 Cooking Time: 20 minutes

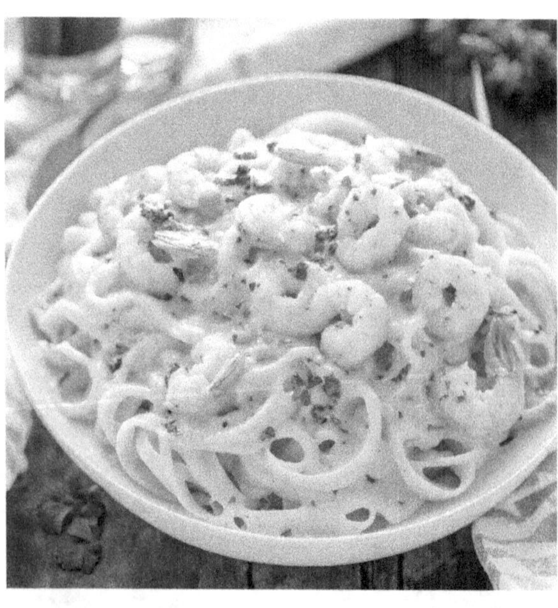

26. Fish Piccata

Ingredients:

- 4 fish fillets (such as tilapia or cod)
- 1/4 cup flour
- 2 tablespoons olive oil
- Juice of 2 lemons
- 1/4 cup capers, drained
- 1/2 cup white wine
- Salt and pepper, to taste
- Fresh parsley, chopped for garnish

Instructions:

1. Season the fish fillets with salt and pepper, then dredge in flour, shaking off the excess.
2. Heat olive oil in a skillet over medium-high heat. Add fish and cook until golden and cooked through, about 3-4 minutes per side.
3. Remove fish from skillet and set aside.
4. Add lemon juice, capers, and white wine to the skillet. Bring to a boil and simmer until the sauce is slightly reduced, about 5 minutes.
5. Return fish to the skillet and warm through.
6. Serve garnished with fresh parsley.

Nutrition Info Per Serving:

- Calories: 260
- Fat: 10g
- Carbohydrates: 8g
- Protein: 30g
- Fiber: 0.5g

Serves: 4 **Cooking Time:** 20 minutes

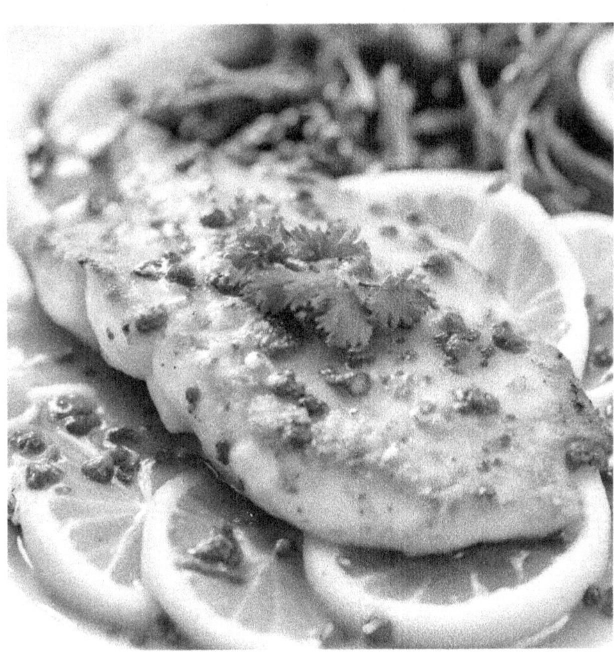

27. Anchovy and Tomato Pasta

Ingredients:
- 1 pound spaghetti
- 2 tablespoons olive oil
- 6 anchovy fillets, minced
- 2 cloves garlic, minced
- 1 can (28 oz) crushed tomatoes
- Red pepper flakes, to taste
- Fresh basil, chopped
- Salt, to taste

Instructions:
1. Cook spaghetti according to package instructions.
2. Heat olive oil in a skillet over medium heat. Add anchovies and garlic, cooking until anchovies dissolve.
3. Stir in crushed tomatoes and red pepper flakes. Simmer for 10 minutes.
4. Season with salt, and mix in fresh basil.
5. Toss the sauce with cooked spaghetti.
6. Serve hot.

Nutrition Info Per Serving:
- Calories: 420
- Fat: 9g
- Carbohydrates: 65g
- Protein: 18g
- Fiber: 4g

Serves: 4 Cooking Time: 20 minutes

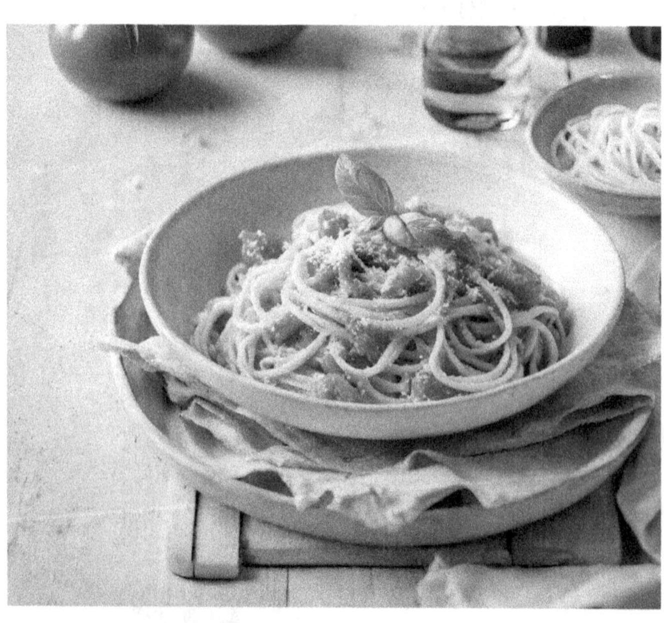

28. Scallop and Pea Risotto

Ingredients:

- 1 pound scallops
- 1 cup Arborio rice
- 1/2 cup peas
- 1 onion, chopped
- 2 cloves garlic, minced
- 4 cups vegetable broth
- 1/2 cup white wine
- 2 tablespoons olive oil
- Salt and pepper, to taste
- Fresh parsley, for garnish

Instructions:

1. Heat 1 tablespoon olive oil in a large skillet over medium heat. Sear scallops for 1-2 minutes per side until golden and just cooked through. Remove and set aside.
2. In the same skillet, add another tablespoon of oil. Add onion and garlic, and sauté until soft.
3. Add Arborio rice, stirring to coat with oil. Pour in white wine and cook until mostly absorbed.
4. Add broth, one cup at a time, stirring frequently, until each addition is absorbed before adding the next.
5. Stir in peas during the last few minutes of cooking.
6. Season with salt and pepper. Serve risotto topped with scallops and garnished with fresh parsley.

Nutrition Info Per Serving:

- Calories: 410
- Fat: 10g
- Carbohydrates: 50g
- Protein: 30g
- Fiber: 3g

Serves: 4 **Cooking Time:** 30 minutes

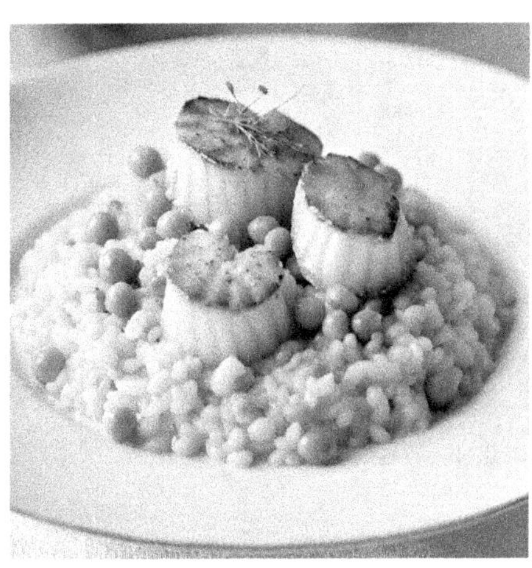

Desserts

1. Grilled Peaches with Cinnamon
Ingredients:
- 4 peaches, halved and pitted
- 2 tablespoons honey
- 1/2 teaspoon ground cinnamon
- Cooking spray or oil for the grill

Instructions:
1. Preheat grill to medium-high heat and lightly oil the grate.
2. Drizzle honey over the cut sides of the peaches and sprinkle with cinnamon.
3. Place peaches, cut side down, on the grill.
4. Grill for 4-5 minutes or until the peaches are tender and have grill marks.
5. Serve warm, optionally with a dollop of Greek yogurt or a sprinkle of crushed nuts.

Nutrition Info Per Serving:
- Calories: 70
- Fat: 0g
- Carbohydrates: 17g
- Protein: 1g
- Fiber: 2g

Serves: 4 **Cooking Time:** 10 minutes

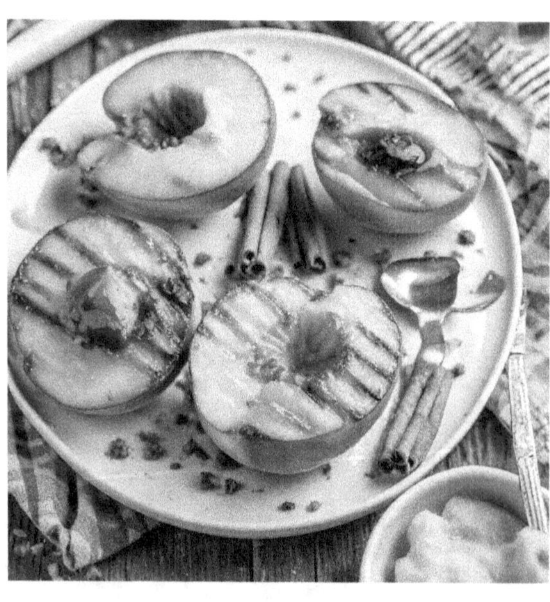

2. Berry Salad with Lemon Drizzle

Ingredients:

- 2 cups mixed berries (strawberries, blueberries, raspberries, blackberries)
- 2 tablespoons honey
- Juice of 1 lemon
- Fresh mint leaves, for garnish

Instructions:

1. In a large bowl, combine the mixed berries.
2. In a small bowl, whisk together honey and lemon juice until well blended.
3. Drizzle the lemon-honey mixture over the berries and toss gently to coat.
4. Garnish with fresh mint leaves before serving.

Nutrition Info Per Serving:

- Calories: 90
- Fat: 0.5g
- Carbohydrates: 22g
- Protein: 1g
- Fiber: 4g

Serves: 4 **Cooking Time:** 5 minutes

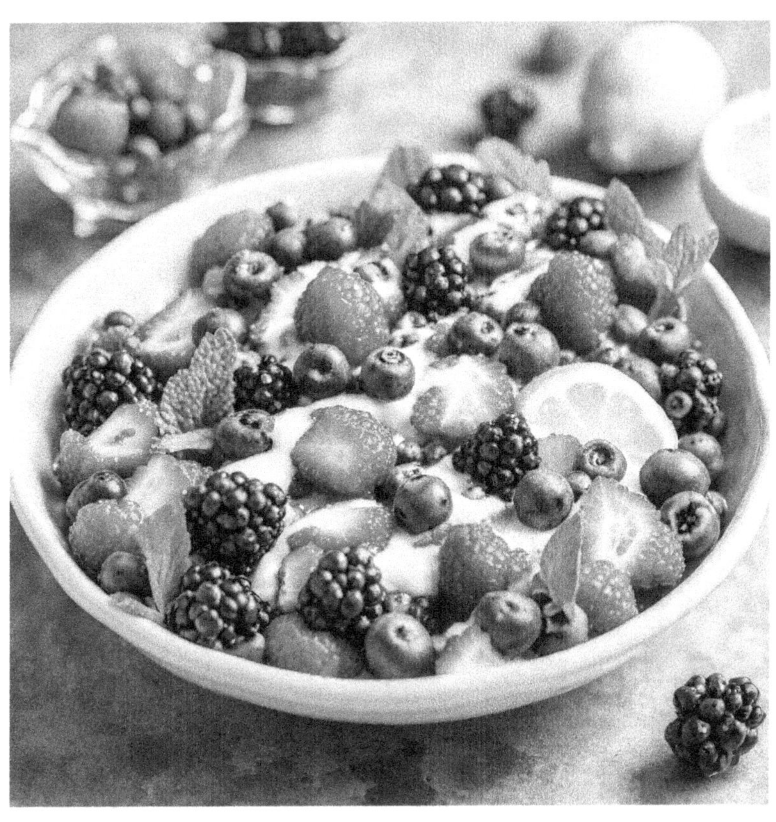

3. Baked Apples with Nut Stuffing

Ingredients:

- 4 large apples, such as Granny Smith or Honeycrisp
- 1/4 cup chopped walnuts
- 1/4 cup almonds, chopped
- 2 tablespoons dried cranberries or raisins
- 1/2 teaspoon ground cinnamon
- 1/4 teaspoon nutmeg
- 2 tablespoons honey
- 1/2 cup apple juice or water

Instructions:

1. Preheat oven to 375°F (190°C).
2. Core the apples, leaving the bottom intact to create a well.
3. In a bowl, mix together walnuts, almonds, cranberries or raisins, cinnamon, and nutmeg.
4. Stuff each apple with the nut mixture and place in a baking dish.
5. Drizzle honey over the stuffed apples.
6. Pour apple juice or water into the bottom of the dish.
7. Bake for 25-30 minutes, or until the apples are tender.
8. Serve warm, spooning the juices over the apples.

Nutrition Info Per Serving:

- Calories: 210
- Fat: 8g
- Carbohydrates: 36g
- Protein: 2g
- Fiber: 5g

Serves: 4 Cooking Time: 30 minutes

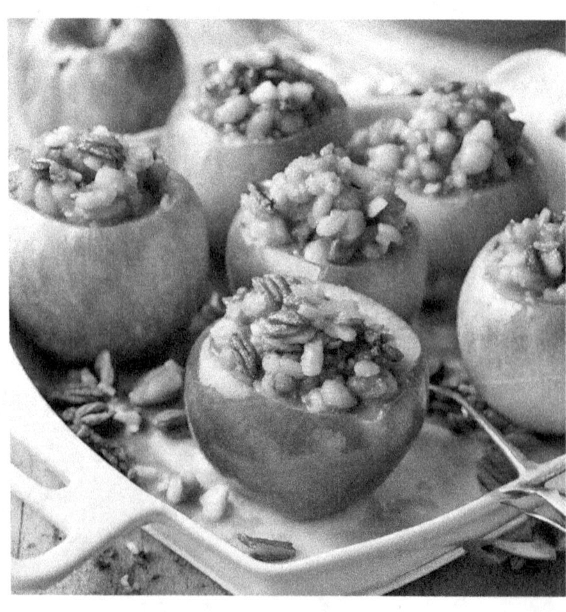

4. Pineapple Carpaccio

Ingredients:

- 1 large pineapple, peeled and cored
- 1 tablespoon honey
- Juice of 1 lime
- Fresh mint leaves, chopped
- A pinch of chili powder (optional)

Instructions:

1. Thinly slice the pineapple into rounds and arrange on a serving plate.
2. In a small bowl, combine honey and lime juice.
3. Drizzle the honey-lime mixture over the pineapple slices.
4. Sprinkle with chopped mint and a pinch of chili powder if using.
5. Chill in the refrigerator for about 10 minutes before serving.

Nutrition Info Per Serving:

- Calories: 120
- Fat: 0g
- Carbohydrates: 32g
- Protein: 1g
- Fiber: 3g

Serves: 4 **Cooking Time:** 15 minutes (including chilling time)

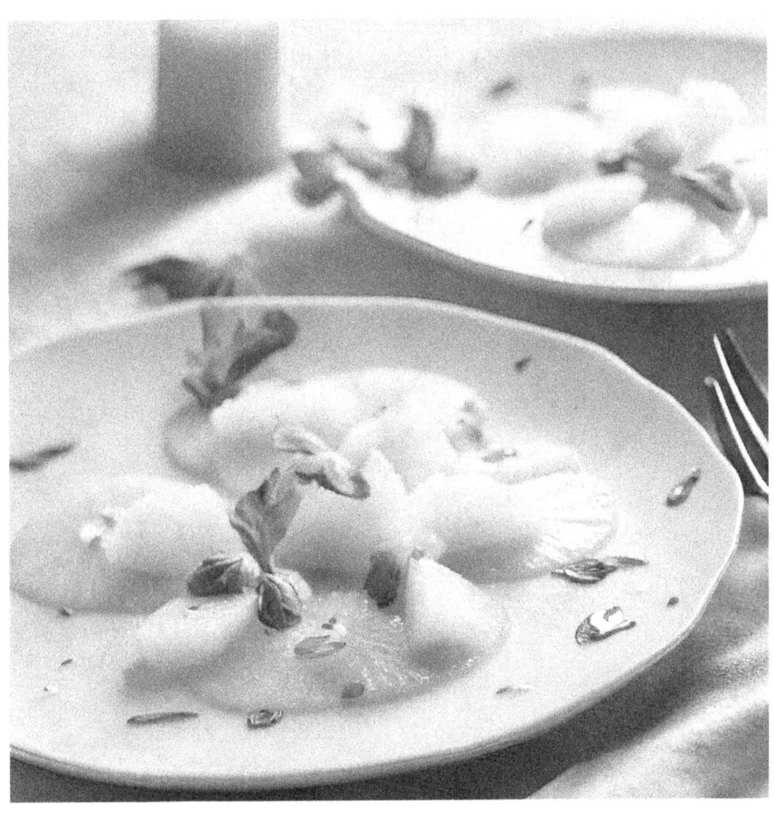

5. Chocolate Avocado Pudding

Ingredients:

- 2 ripe avocados, peeled and pitted
- 1/4 cup cocoa powder
- 1/4 cup honey or maple syrup
- 1/2 cup coconut milk
- 1 teaspoon vanilla extract
- Pinch of salt

Instructions:

1. Combine avocados, cocoa powder, honey, coconut milk, vanilla extract, and salt in a blender.
2. Blend until smooth, scraping down the sides as necessary.
3. Chill in the refrigerator for at least 15 minutes before serving.
4. Serve chilled with a sprinkle of grated chocolate or fresh berries.

Nutrition Info Per Serving:

- Calories: 250
- Fat: 15g
- Carbohydrates: 30g
- Protein: 3g
- Fiber: 7g

Serves: 4 **Cooking Time:** 15 minutes

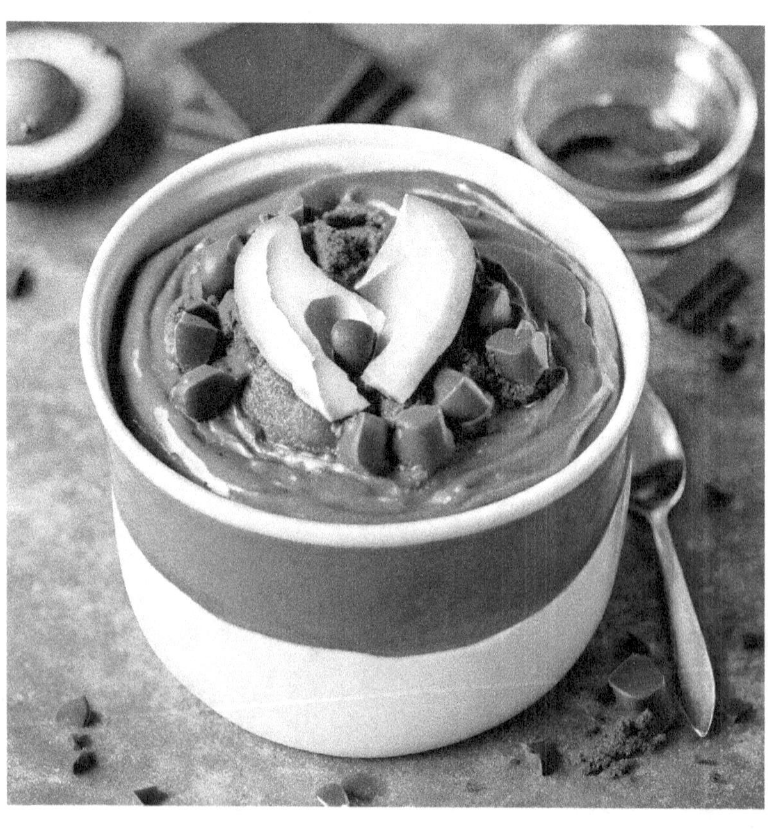

6. Nut Butter Cups

Ingredients:

- 1 cup dark chocolate chips
- 1/2 cup peanut or almond butter
- 2 tablespoons honey
- 1/4 teaspoon sea salt
- Mini muffin liners

Instructions:

1. Melt chocolate chips in a microwave-safe bowl or double boiler until smooth.
2. Line a mini muffin tin with liners and spoon a layer of melted chocolate into each.
3. Freeze for 5 minutes to set.
4. Mix nut butter with honey and salt. Spoon a small amount into each chocolate base.
5. Cover with more melted chocolate and smooth the tops.
6. Freeze for another 15 minutes until set.
7. Keep refrigerated until ready to serve.

Nutrition Info Per Serving:

- Calories: 150
- Fat: 10g
- Carbohydrates: 12g
- Protein: 4g
- Fiber: 1g

Serves: 12 cups **Cooking Time:** 20 minutes

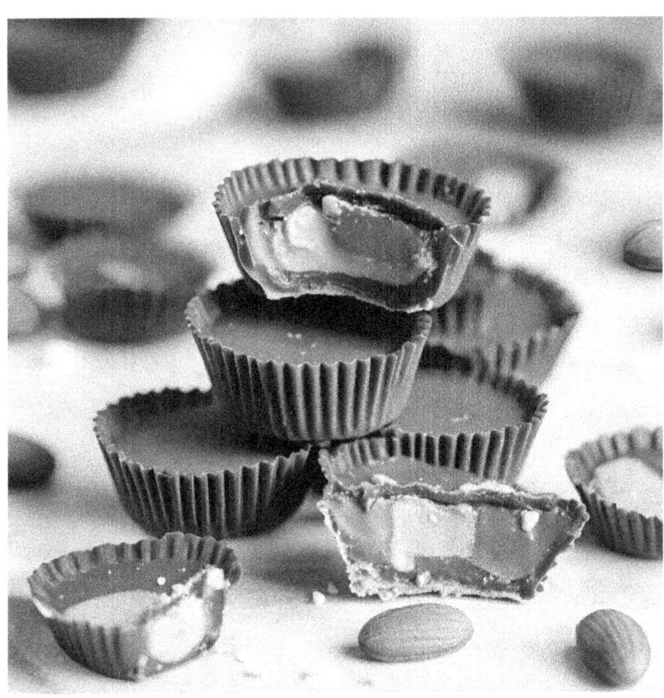

7. Coconut Balls

Ingredients:

- 2 cups shredded unsweetened coconut
- 1/2 cup almond flour
- 1/3 cup maple syrup
- 1/4 cup coconut oil, melted
- 1 teaspoon vanilla extract

Instructions:

1. In a bowl, mix all ingredients until well combined.
2. Roll the mixture into small balls and place on a baking sheet lined with parchment paper.
3. Freeze for about 15 minutes or until firm.
4. Store in an airtight container in the refrigerator.

Nutrition Info Per Serving:

- Calories: 130
- Fat: 10g
- Carbohydrates: 10g
- Protein: 1g
- Fiber: 2g

Serves: 12 Cooking Time: 15 minutes

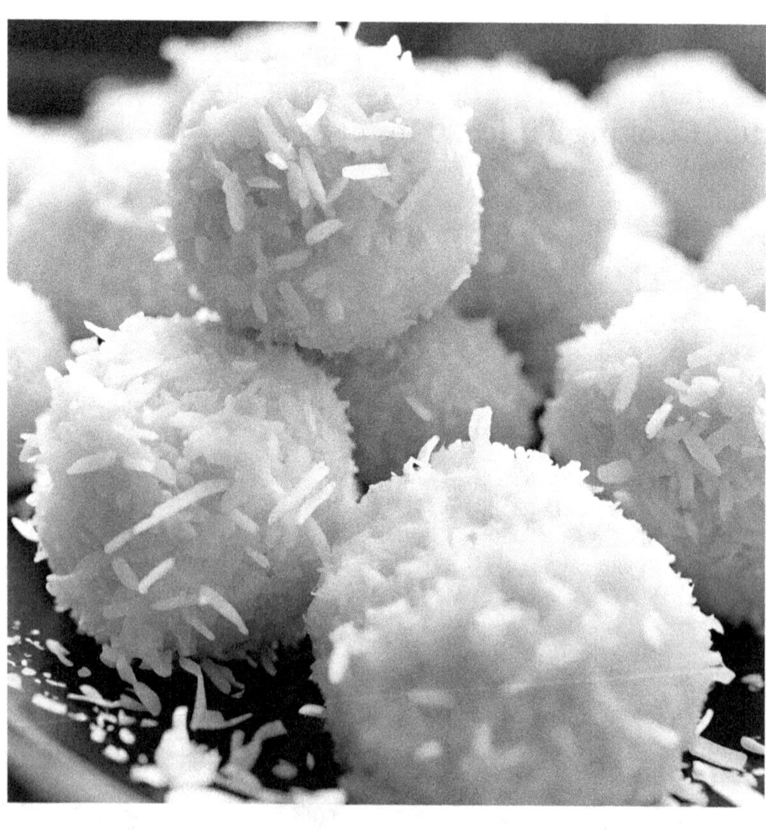

8. Almond Joy Bars

Ingredients:

- 1 cup shredded unsweetened coconut
- 1/3 cup condensed coconut milk
- 1/4 cup slivered almonds
- 1 cup dark chocolate chips, melted

Instructions:

1. In a bowl, mix coconut and condensed coconut milk until well combined.
2. Press the mixture into a small lined baking dish.
3. Sprinkle slivered almonds over the top and press gently into the coconut base.
4. Pour melted chocolate over the almonds and spread evenly.
5. Refrigerate until set, about 20 minutes. Cut into bars and serve.

Nutrition Info Per Serving:

- Calories: 200
- Fat: 15g
- Carbohydrates: 15g
- Protein: 3g
- Fiber: 3g

Serves: 8 **Cooking Time:** 25 minutes

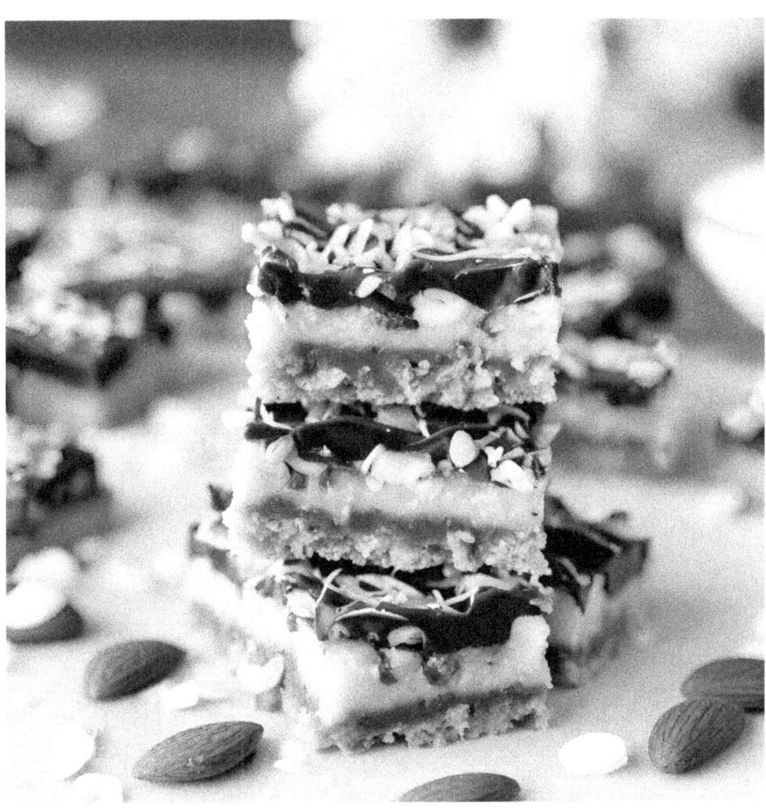

9. Almond Flour Shortbread Cookies

Ingredients:

- 2 cups almond flour
- 1/3 cup softened coconut oil
- 1/3 cup maple syrup
- 1 teaspoon vanilla extract
- Pinch of salt

Instructions:

1. Preheat oven to 350°F (175°C).
2. In a bowl, mix all ingredients until a dough forms.
3. Roll the dough into balls and press down slightly to form cookies on a lined baking sheet.
4. Bake for 12-15 minutes or until edges are golden.
5. Let cool on the sheet for 10 minutes before transferring to a wire rack.

Nutrition Info Per Serving:

- Calories: 160
- Fat: 12g
- Carbohydrates: 10g
- Protein: 4g
- Fiber: 2g

Serves: 12 **Cooking Time:** 15 minutes

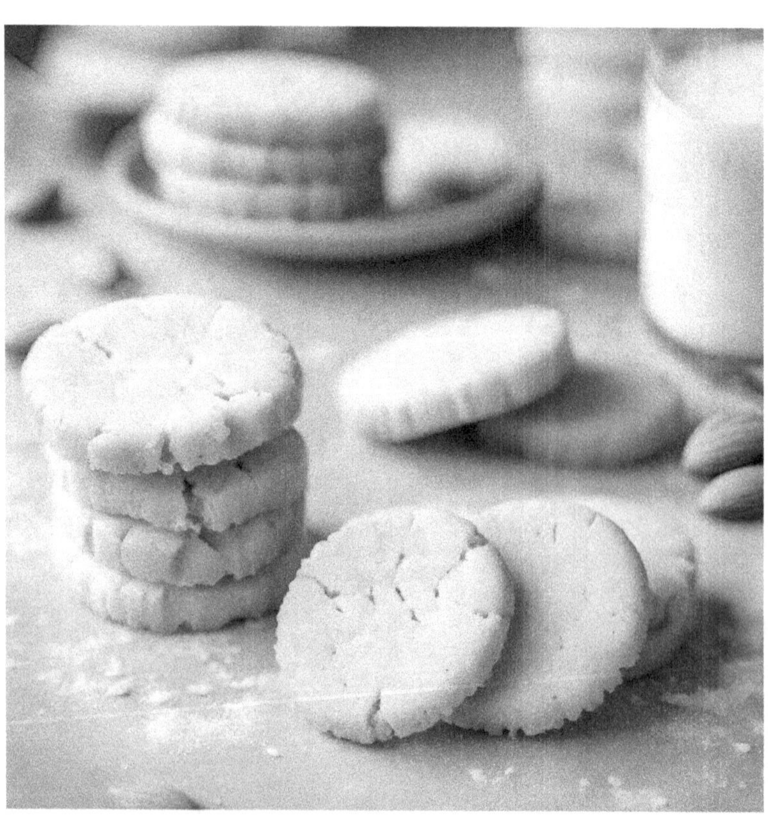

10. Pumpkin Spice Muffins
Ingredients:
- 2 cups almond flour
- 1/2 cup canned pumpkin
- 1/3 cup maple syrup
- 2 eggs
- 1 teaspoon baking powder
- 1 teaspoon cinnamon
- 1/2 teaspoon nutmeg
- 1/4 teaspoon cloves
- Pinch of salt

Instructions:
1. Preheat oven to 350°F (175°C).
2. In a bowl, combine all ingredients and mix until smooth.
3. Divide the batter among lined muffin cups.
4. Bake for 18-20 minutes or until a toothpick comes out clean.
5. Let cool before serving.

Nutrition Info Per Serving:
- Calories: 150
- Fat: 10g
- Carbohydrates: 12g
- Protein: 5g
- Fiber: 3g

Serves: 12 muffins **Cooking Time:** 20 minutes

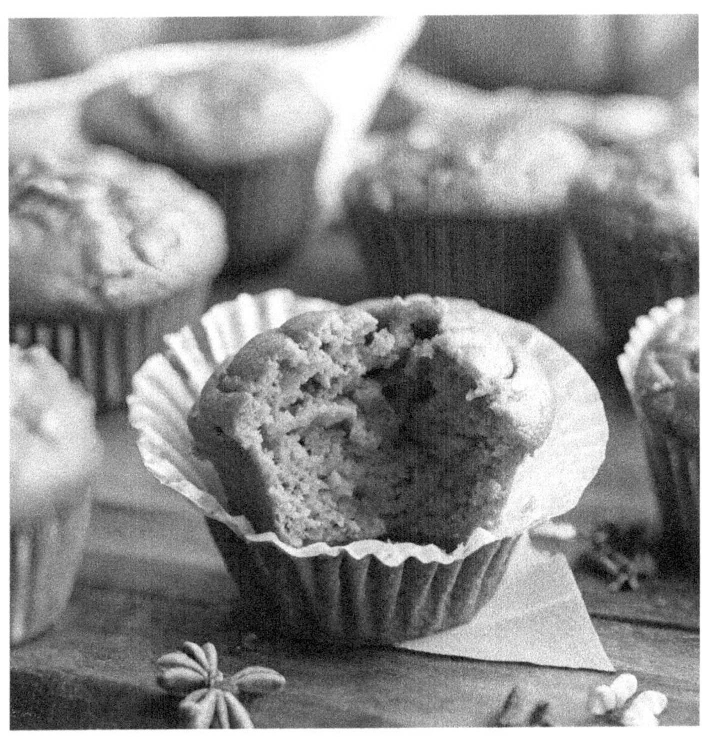

11. Lemon Ricotta Cookies
Ingredients:
- 2 cups almond flour
- 1/2 cup ricotta cheese
- 1/4 cup honey
- Zest of 1 lemon
- 1 teaspoon vanilla extract

Instructions:
1. Preheat oven to 350°F (175°C).
2. In a bowl, mix all ingredients until a cohesive dough forms.
3. Drop spoonfuls of dough onto a lined baking sheet and flatten slightly.
4. Bake for 12-15 minutes or until the edges are golden.
5. Let cool on the sheet before transferring to a rack.

Nutrition Info Per Serving:
- Calories: 180
- Fat: 14g
- Carbohydrates: 10g
- Protein: 5g
- Fiber: 2g

Serves: 12 cookies **Cooking Time:** 15 minutes

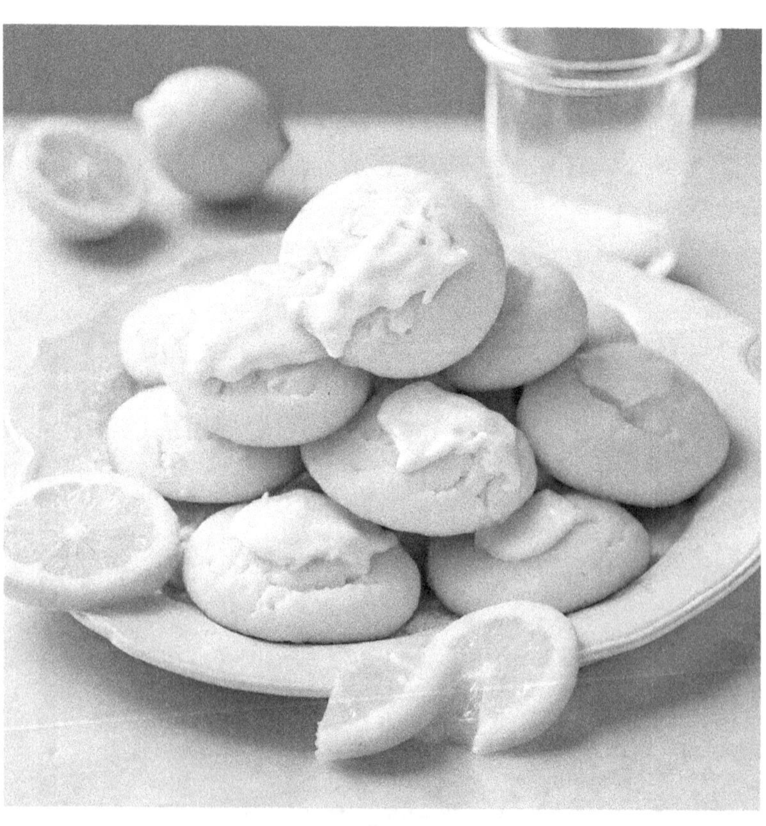

12. Zucchini Brownies

Ingredients:

- 1 medium zucchini, grated
- 1 cup almond flour
- 1/2 cup cocoa powder
- 1/4 cup coconut oil, melted
- 1/4 cup honey
- 2 eggs
- 1 teaspoon vanilla extract
- 1/2 teaspoon baking powder
- Pinch of salt

Instructions:

1. Preheat oven to 350°F (175°C).
2. Squeeze excess moisture from the grated zucchini using a cloth.
3. In a bowl, mix zucchini with all other ingredients until well combined.
4. Pour into a greased 8x8 inch baking dish.
5. Bake for 20-25 minutes or until a toothpick comes out mostly clean.
6. Let cool before cutting into squares and serving.

Nutrition Info Per Serving:

- Calories: 150
- Fat: 11g
- Carbohydrates: 12g
- Protein: 4g
- Fiber: 3g

Serves: 16 brownies **Cooking Time:** 25 minutes

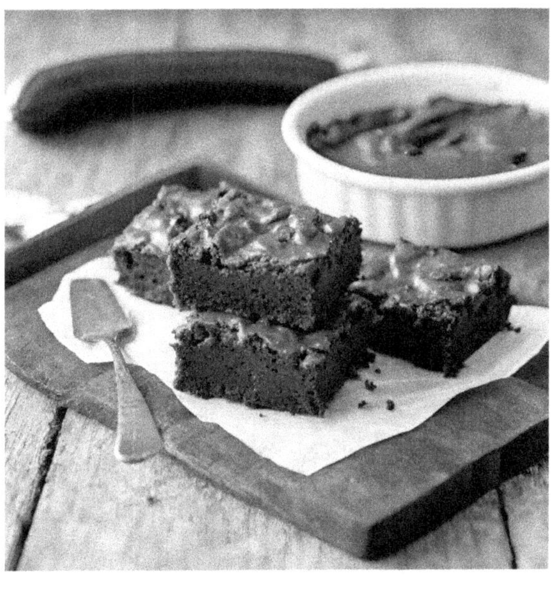

13. Indian Rice Pudding (Kheer)

Ingredients:

- 1/2 cup basmati rice
- 4 cups milk (use almond milk for a dairy-free option)
- 1/4 cup sugar
- 1/2 teaspoon ground cardamom
- 1/4 cup raisins
- 1/4 cup chopped almonds
- A pinch of saffron (optional)

Instructions:

1. Rinse the rice under cold water until the water runs clear.
2. In a large saucepan, combine the rice, milk, and saffron. Bring to a boil, then reduce heat to low and simmer, stirring occasionally, until the rice is soft and the mixture has thickened, about 20-25 minutes.
3. Add sugar, cardamom, raisins, and almonds. Cook for another 5 minutes.
4. Remove from heat and let cool slightly. Serve warm or chilled, garnished with more nuts if desired.

Nutrition Info Per Serving:

- Calories: 220
- Fat: 5g
- Carbohydrates: 38g
- Protein: 6g
- Fiber: 1g

Serves: 4 **Cooking Time:** 30 minutes

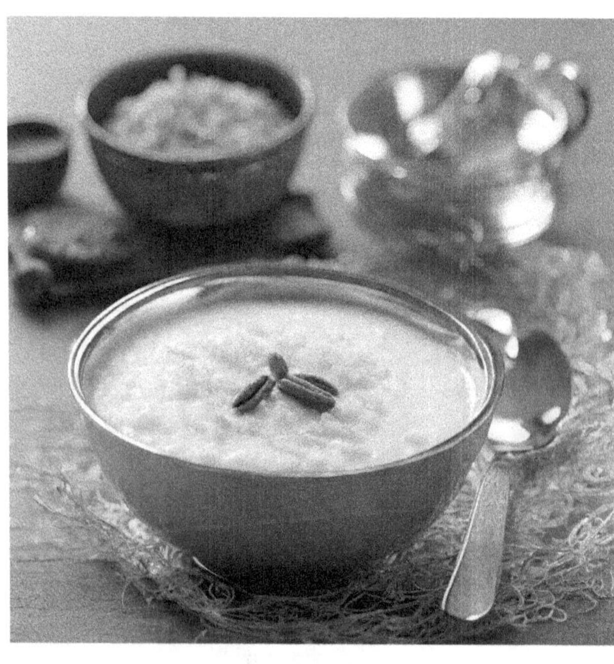

14. Italian Affogato

Ingredients:

- 4 scoops vanilla ice cream (use coconut or almond milk ice cream for a dairy-free option)
- 2 shots espresso or 1/2 cup strong brewed coffee

Instructions:

1. Place a scoop of ice cream in each serving glass.
2. Pour a shot of hot espresso or 1/4 cup of hot brewed coffee over each ice cream scoop.
3. Serve immediately, allowing the ice cream to melt slightly into the coffee for a creamy dessert.

Nutrition Info Per Serving:

- Calories: 170
- Fat: 9g
- Carbohydrates: 20g
- Protein: 3g
- Fiber: 0g

Serves: 4 **Cooking Time:** 5 minutes

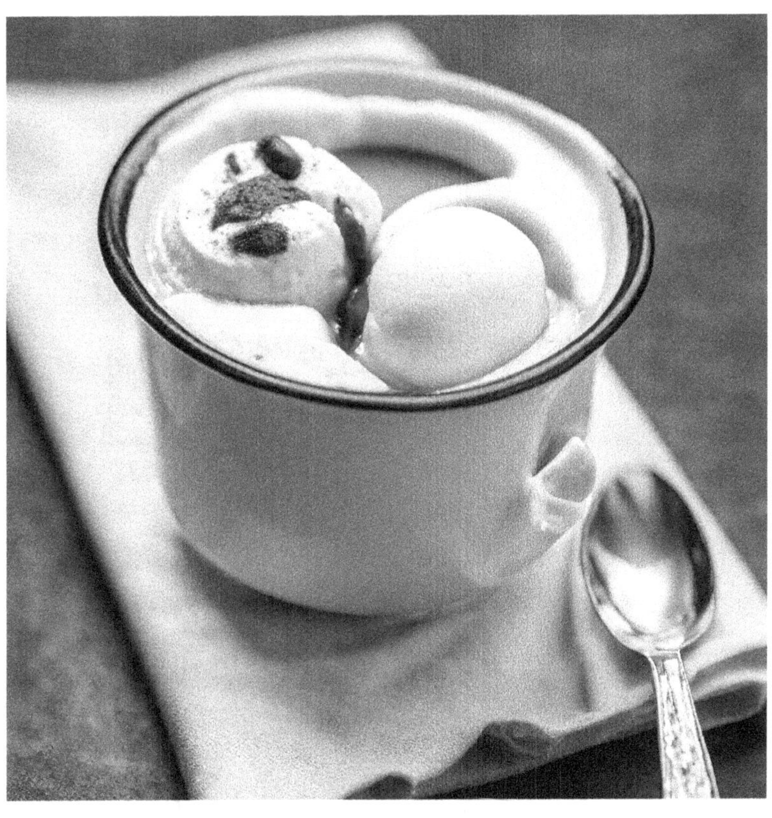

15. Turkish Halva

Ingredients:
- 1 cup fine semolina
- 1/2 cup sugar
- 1/2 cup unsalted butter
- 2 cups water
- 1/2 teaspoon ground cinnamon
- 1/4 cup pine nuts or chopped pistachios

Instructions:
1. In a saucepan, bring water and sugar to a boil until sugar is dissolved. Set aside.
2. In another pan, melt butter over medium heat. Add semolina and cook, stirring constantly, until golden brown, about 5-7 minutes.
3. Slowly pour the sugar syrup over the semolina mixture, stirring constantly. Continue to cook until the mixture thickens and starts to pull away from the sides of the pan.
4. Stir in cinnamon and pine nuts or pistachios.
5. Pour halva into a mold or dish and let set for about 20 minutes before slicing and serving.

Nutrition Info Per Serving:
- Calories: 450
- Fat: 25g
- Carbohydrates: 52g
- Protein: 6g
- Fiber: 2g

Serves: 4 **Cooking Time:** 25 minutes

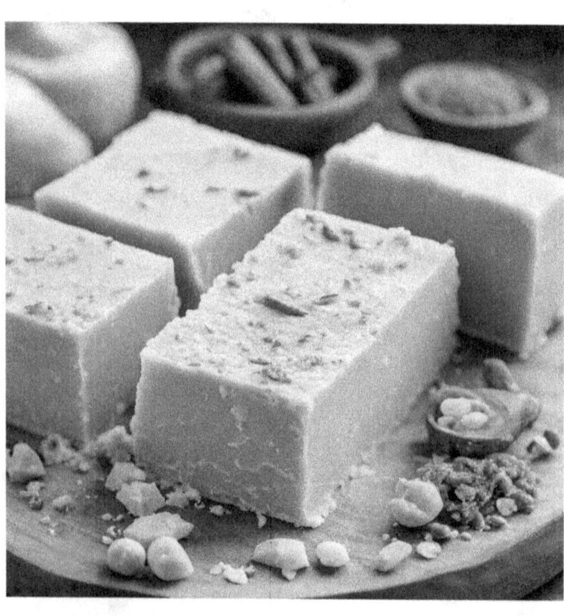

16. Mini Pavlovas

Ingredients:

- 4 egg whites
- 1 cup granulated sugar
- 1 teaspoon vanilla extract
- 1 teaspoon white vinegar
- 1 tablespoon cornstarch
- Toppings: Whipped cream, fresh berries, and mint leaves

Instructions:

1. Preheat oven to 250°F (120°C). Line a baking sheet with parchment paper.
2. In a clean bowl, beat egg whites until soft peaks form. Gradually add sugar, beating until stiff peaks form.
3. Fold in vanilla extract, vinegar, and cornstarch.
4. Spoon the meringue into small rounds on the prepared baking sheet.
5. Bake for 50-60 minutes, or until the pavlovas are dry to the touch. Turn off the oven and let them cool inside.
6. Top with whipped cream, fresh berries, and mint before serving.

Nutrition Info Per Serving:

- Calories: 210
- Fat: 6g
- Carbohydrates: 38g
- Protein: 2g
- Fiber: 1g

Serves: 4 **Cooking Time:** 60 minutes

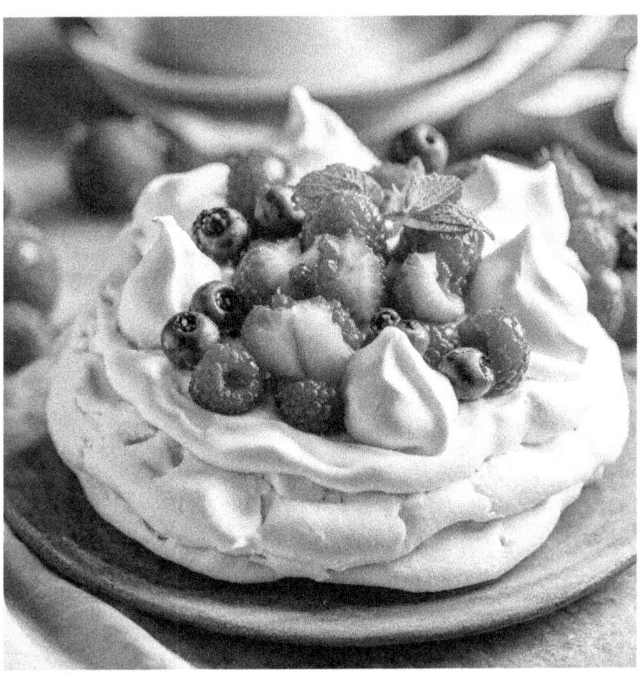

17. Mini Key Lime Pies
Ingredients:

- 1 cup graham cracker crumbs (use gluten-free if necessary)
- 1/4 cup melted butter
- 1/4 cup sugar for crust
- 1 can (14 oz) condensed milk (use coconut condensed milk for dairy-free)
- 1/2 cup key lime juice
- 2 teaspoons lime zest
- 1/4 cup sugar for filling

Instructions:

1. Preheat oven to 350°F (175°C).
2. Mix graham cracker crumbs, melted butter, and 1/4 cup sugar. Press into mini tart pans or a muffin tin to form the crusts.
3. In a bowl, combine condensed milk, lime juice, lime zest, and 1/4 cup sugar. Mix until smooth.
4. Pour the filling into the crusts and bake for 10-12 minutes until set.
5. Chill in the refrigerator for at least 1 hour before serving.

Nutrition Info Per Serving:

- Calories: 320
- Fat: 12g
- Carbohydrates: 50g
- Protein: 5g
- Fiber: 0g

Serves: 4 Cooking Time: 20 minutes (plus chilling)

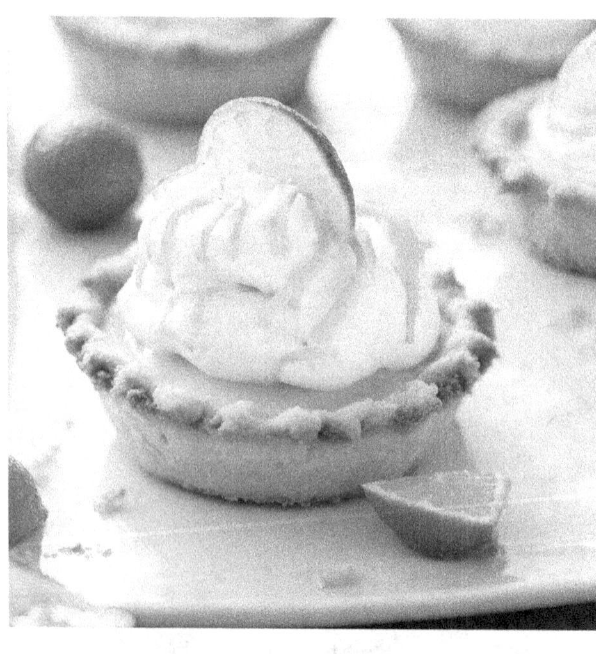

6-WEEK MEAL PLAN

Week 1

Day 1:
- **Breakfast:** Pear and Walnut Salad
- **Lunch:** Cucumber and Herb Salad with Feta
- **Dinner:** Grilled Mackerel with Herbs

Day 2:
- **Breakfast:** Ricotta and Berry Tarts
- **Lunch:** Nutty Yogurt Bowl
- **Dinner:** Beef and Broccoli Stir-Fry

Day 3:
- **Breakfast:** Melon and Prosciutto Plate
- **Lunch:** Breakfast Veggie Pockets
- **Dinner:** Lemon Herb Chicken Breast

Day 4:
- **Breakfast:** Greek Yogurt Parfait
- **Lunch:** Turkey and Spinach Breakfast Hash
- **Dinner:** Turkey Cobb Salad

Day 5:
- **Breakfast:** Sardine Salad
- **Lunch:** Tomato and Olive Tapenade on Toast
- **Dinner:** Quick Fish Stew

Day 6:
- **Breakfast:** Smoked Turkey and Avocado Sandwich
- **Lunch:** Cottage Cheese and Pineapple Toast
- **Dinner:** Pan-Seared Duck Breast

Day 7:
- **Breakfast:** Almond Butter and Banana Sandwich
- **Lunch:** Avocado and Radish Toast
- **Dinner:** Thai Coconut Curry Chicken

Week 2

Day 8:
- **Breakfast:** Creamy Millet Porridge
- **Lunch:** Warm Buckwheat Bowl
- **Dinner:** Moroccan Grilled Fish

Day 9:
- **Breakfast:** Quinoa Porridge with Almonds
- **Lunch:** Chia and Lemon Pancakes
- **Dinner:** Asian-Style Tuna Steaks

Day 11:
- **Breakfast:** Coconut Flour Waffles
- **Lunch:** Greek Salad with Grilled Chicken
- **Dinner:** Quick Beef Stroganoff

Day 12:
- **Breakfast:** Almond Flour Pancakes
- **Lunch:** Sunny-Side Hemp Seeds
- **Dinner:** Garlic Herb Pork Chops

Day 13:
- **Breakfast:** Tomato Avocado Egg Muffins
- **Lunch:** Kale and Quinoa Salad
- **Dinner:** Moroccan Spiced Meatballs

Day 14:
- **Breakfast:** Iodine-Rich Seaweed Smoothie
- **Lunch:** Spinach and Avocado Salad
- **Dinner:** Garlic Lemon Mussels

Week 3

Day 15:
- **Breakfast:** Berry Selenium Boost Smoothie
- **Lunch:** Spinach and White Bean Soup
- **Dinner:** Pan-Fried Calamari with Aioli

Day 16:
- **Breakfast:** Grilled Peaches with Cinnamon
- **Lunch:** Roasted Red Pepper Soup
- **Dinner:** Shrimp and Avocado Taco Salad

Day 17:
- **Breakfast:** Berry Salad with Lemon Drizzle
- **Lunch:** Butternut Squash Soup
- **Dinner:** Lobster Tail with Herb Butter

Day 18:
- **Breakfast:** Baked Apples with Nut Stuffing
- **Lunch:** Chicken Zoodle Soup
- **Dinner:** Oyster Mushroom Ceviche

Day 19:
- **Breakfast:** Pineapple Carpaccio
- **Lunch:** Creamy Avocado Cucumber Soup
- **Dinner:** Fish Piccata

Day 20:
- **Breakfast:** Chocolate Avocado Pudding
- **Lunch:** Beet and Ginger Soup
- **Dinner:** Anchovy and Tomato Pasta

Day 21:
- **Breakfast:** Nut Butter Cups
- **Lunch:** Miso Soup with Mushrooms
- **Dinner:** Scallop and Pea Risotto

Week 4

Day 22:
- **Breakfast:** Coconut Balls
- **Lunch:** Broccoli and Bacon Salad
- **Dinner:** Italian Herbed Steak

Day 23:
- **Breakfast:** Almond Joy Bars
- **Lunch:** Shrimp and Avocado Salad
- **Dinner:** Meatloaf Muffins

Day 24:
- **Breakfast:** Almond Flour Shortbread Cookies
- **Lunch:** Endive and Apple Salad
- **Dinner:** Spicy Ground Lamb with Peas

Day 25:
- **Breakfast:** Pumpkin Spice Muffins
- **Lunch:** Carrot and Raisin Salad
- **Dinner:** Chicken and Beef Kabobs

Day 26:
- **Breakfast:** Lemon Ricotta Cookies
- **Lunch:** Radish and Spring Onion Salad
- **Dinner:** Herb-Roasted Turkey Breast

Day 27:
- **Breakfast:** Zucchini Brownies
- **Lunch:** Broccoli Almond Soup
- **Dinner:** Mediterranean Lamb Salad

Day 28:
- **Breakfast:** Indian Rice Pudding (Kheer)
- **Lunch:** Asian Chicken Salad
- **Dinner:** Tuna Salad Nicoise

Week 5

Day 29:
- **Breakfast:** Italian Affogato
- **Lunch:** Turkey Cobb Salad
- **Dinner:** Mini Pavlovas

Day 30:
- **Breakfast:** Turkish Halva
- **Lunch:** Beetroot and Goat Cheese Salad
- **Dinner:** Mini Key Lime Pies

Day 31:
- **Breakfast:** Lemon Garlic Tilapia
- **Lunch:** Herb-Crusted Salmon
- **Dinner:** Garlic Butter Shrimp

Day 32:
- **Breakfast:** Honey Mustard Cod
- **Lunch:** Mediterranean Sardine Salad
- **Dinner:** Pesto Shrimp Skewers

Day 33:
- **Breakfast:** Seared Scallops with Lemon Sauce
- **Lunch:** Smoked Salmon Breakfast Wrap
- **Dinner:** Grilled Mackerel with Herbs

Day 34:
- **Breakfast:** Clam Chowder (Dairy-Free)
- **Lunch:** Crab Salad with Citrus Vinaigrette
- **Dinner:** Thai Coconut Shrimp Soup

Day 35:
- **Breakfast:** Garlic Lemon Mussels
- **Lunch:** Pan-Fried Calamari with Aioli
- **Dinner:** Shrimp and Avocado Taco Salad

Week 6

Day 36:
- **Breakfast:** Lobster Tail with Herb Butter
- **Lunch:** Oyster Mushroom Ceviche
- **Dinner:** Baked Clams with Garlic

Day 37:
- **Breakfast:** Scallops with Asparagus
- **Lunch:** Moroccan Grilled Fish
- **Dinner:** Asian-Style Tuna Steaks

Day 38:
- **Breakfast:** Indian-Spiced Shrimp Curry
- **Lunch:** Greek-Style Baked Sardines
- **Dinner:** Quick Fish Stew

Day 39:
- **Breakfast:** Shrimp Alfredo (Dairy-Free)
- **Lunch:** Fish Piccata
- **Dinner:** Anchovy and Tomato Pasta

Day 40:
- **Breakfast:** Scallop and Pea Risotto
- **Lunch:** Chocolate Avocado Pudding
- **Dinner:** Nut Butter Cups

Day 41:
- **Breakfast:** Coconut Balls
- **Lunch:** Almond Joy Bars
- **Dinner:** Almond Flour Shortbread Cookies

Day 42:
- **Breakfast:** Pumpkin Spice Muffins
- **Lunch:** Lemon Ricotta Cookies
- **Dinner:** Zucchini Brownies

WEEKLY MEAL PLANNER 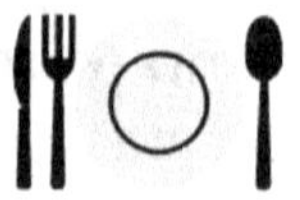

	BREAKFAST	LUNCH	DINNER	SNACKS
MONDAY				
TUESDAY				
WEDNESDAY				
THURSDAY				
FRIDAY				
SATURDAY				
SUNDAY				

What symptoms of thyroid disease have been most challenging for you? How do they affect your daily life?

WEEKLY MEAL PLANNER

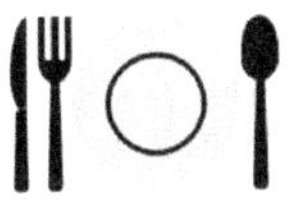

	BREAKFAST	LUNCH	DINNER	SNACKS
MONDAY				
TUESDAY				
WEDNESDAY				
THURSDAY				
FRIDAY				
SATURDAY				
SUNDAY				

Before starting the thyroid diet, what do you already know about how diet affects thyroid health?

WEEKLY MEAL PLANNER

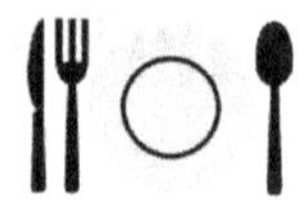

	BREAKFAST	LUNCH	DINNER	SNACKS
MONDAY				
TUESDAY				
WEDNESDAY				
THURSDAY				
FRIDAY				
SATURDAY				
SUNDAY				

What are your main health goals for starting the thyroid diet? Are you looking to improve energy, lose weight, or stabilize your thyroid levels?

WEEKLY MEAL PLANNER 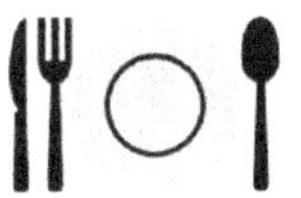

	BREAKFAST	LUNCH	DINNER	SNACKS
MONDAY				
TUESDAY				
WEDNESDAY				
THURSDAY				
FRIDAY				
SATURDAY				
SUNDAY				

Have you tried any other diets or lifestyle changes in the past to manage your thyroid condition? What were the results?

WEEKLY MEAL PLANNER 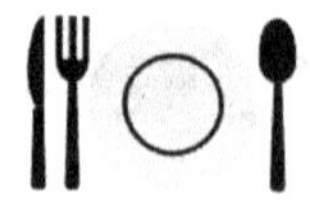

	BREAKFAST	LUNCH	DINNER	SNACKS
MONDAY				
TUESDAY				
WEDNESDAY				
THURSDAY				
FRIDAY				
SATURDAY				
SUNDAY				

What are your expectations from the thyroid diet? How do you think this approach will be different from your previous experiences?

WEEKLY MEAL PLANNER 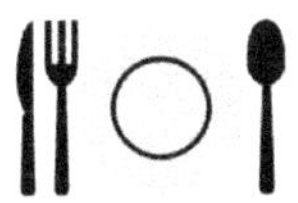

	BREAKFAST	LUNCH	DINNER	SNACKS
MONDAY				
TUESDAY				
WEDNESDAY				
THURSDAY				
FRIDAY				
SATURDAY				
SUNDAY				

Which foods do you understand to be particularly beneficial or harmful for thyroid health?
How do you feel about adjusting your diet to incorporate more thyroid-supporting foods?

WEEKLY MEAL PLANNER 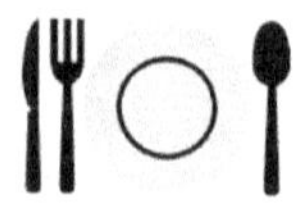

	BREAKFAST	LUNCH	DINNER	SNACKS
MONDAY				
TUESDAY				
WEDNESDAY				
THURSDAY				
FRIDAY				
SATURDAY				
SUNDAY				

How will you handle situations where non-thyroid-friendly foods are in abundance, such as at parties or family gatherings?

WEEKLY MEAL PLANNER

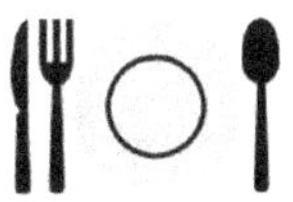

	BREAKFAST	LUNCH	DINNER	SNACKS
MONDAY				
TUESDAY				
WEDNESDAY				
THURSDAY				
FRIDAY				
SATURDAY				
SUNDAY				

What would you like to have learned about yourself and your health after three months on the thyroid diet?

Please Scan this QR Code to Get Your Bonus Content